Edgar Cayce's

Quick & Easy

Remedies

Edgar Cayce's

Quick & Easy
Remedies

A Holistic Guide to Healing Packs,
Poultices, and Other Homemade Remedies

Elaine Hruska

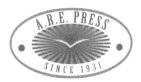

A.R.E. Press • Virginia Beach • Virginia

A.R.E. Press
215 67th Street
Virginia Beach, VA 23451-2061

ISBN 13: 978-0-87604-627-2

Cover design by Christine Fulcher

CONTENTS

Introduction

We spend annually billions of dollars on over-the-counter health remedies to take care of minor emergencies, aching muscles, scratches, sores, or illnesses deemed too minor to warrant a physician's office visit—not realizing that in many cases some of these remedies can be found in the home cupboard, kitchen pantry, or closet, within easy access to us. Such is the case with a number of the recommended treatments in the readings of Edgar Cayce (1877-1945), considered to be America's best-documented psychic. Cayce left over 9,000 individual health readings (out of more than 14,000) that continue to be studied and analyzed for their useful information on various illnesses.

This book is an attempt to present some of these home remedies in an easy-to-use format, introducing the reader to the individual item while noting the symptoms for each one (indications) and also the contraindications (if any). The text will present the various treatments (as given in the readings) and how often, how long, and how much to use, as well as the expected effects or results. Directions are included along with selected excerpts from the readings and some testimonials from individuals who used the remedy.

For individuals new to or unfamiliar with the Cayce readings, it is helpful to note that the language of the readings is at times challenging to comprehend; this difficulty seems to be particularly true with the physical readings. Cayce's explanation of health and his descriptions of the workings of the physical body encompass a holistic approach. Additionally, he often seems to use anatomical terms in a somewhat different way from current usage. To a large extent throughout the book, this language, at times paraphrased, is used in the descriptions of the information presented in these chapters. (*See also* **A Note to the Reader** for an explanation of the reading numbers and other designations from the readings.) Though the excerpts may require several re-reads to grasp their meaning, the effort to comprehend them is worth the struggle as new insights are born and fresh perspectives are challenged. It is hoped that what is presented here is useful and beneficial, contributing greatly to your overall health and wellness.

A Note to the Reader: The number following the excerpt represents the recipient of the reading—each individual was assigned a number to provide anonymity. The first set of numbers refers to the individual or group who received the reading; the second set represents its place in a sequence. For example, in reading 294-3, "294" stands for the person's name, while "-3" represents the third reading given for that individual.

When the readings were computerized, the body of the reading was referred to as the "text." Any notes, letters, background information, related articles, etc., were also placed alongside the text of the reading. Stylistically, "B" means background and "R" means reports. To locate this information more easily, these letters were used. For example, "202-1, Report #5" means that in reading 202-1, under reports (R), item number 5, can be found that particular quote or information.

It is important to remember that the readings were given for individuals even though they carry a universality of content. With the physical readings, however, it should be noted that the information is not meant to be used for self-diagnosis or self-treatment. Any medical problems need the supervision and advice of a health care professional.

Apple Cider Vinegar (and Salt) Pack

A pack is any type of wrapping such as a blanket, sheet, or towel—wet or dry or hot or cold—placed around the whole person or a limb, or it may be a simple compress applied to a body area. Because of the addition of apple cider vinegar (and/or salt) to the compress, this pack is technically a stupe.

For this remedy there are several types of application. Pour the vinegar by itself onto a towel and place it on the skin. Or you may add salt to this compress. Or make a paste by dampening the salt with the vinegar and massaging it into the area. Or create a salt pack, using a pillow; heat the salt and pour it into the pillow, then place it, like a heating pad, onto the vinegar–soaked towel. Sometimes vinegar is also added to dampen the salt in the pillow. (See *Directions* for more detailed instructions.)

What are the effects of the salt and vinegar combination? " . . . The reaction of this acid with the sodium chloride is to produce to the system a drawing from the glands and from the soft tissue of the body those poisons in the form of a perspiration . . . " (829-1) Accordingly, a detoxifying effect is produced in the body by this application.

Vinegar, a beloved staple domestic item, was used as an antibiotic and antiseptic in ancient times by the Egyptians, Greeks, and Romans. It can be found in approximately ninety-eight percent of American homes, mainly in the form of distilled white vinegar or apple cider vinegar. If produced from whole, good-quality apples not treated with toxic chemicals, the vinegar contains healthy enzymes, amino acids, vitamins, and minerals.

The Cayce readings mention apple cider vinegar (frequently named "apple vinegar") in over one hundred documents, recommending it as an application for local massages and packs (usually combined with salt), for sunburn, in baths, and as an ingredient in a hair rinse (one reading).

INDICATIONS

Adhesions, arthritis, broken bones, bruised tendons, cartilage misalignment, colitis, fingernails, fractures, injuries, joint pain, lesions, lumbago, neuritis, pelvic cellulitis, rheumatism, spinal misalignments, sprains, strains, sunburn, torn ligaments, tuberculosis (bone), vulvitis

CONTRAINDICATIONS

Check for skin sensitivity to vinegar by applying a small amount to an area of skin; wait a few minutes for any reaction such as a rash or redness; do not use if a reaction occurs.

MATERIALS NEEDED

Apple cider vinegar—organic, if available [" . . . not that which is synthetically made . . . " (404-14)]

One or two pillowcases—if making a salt pack

Several towels or washcloths—to use as compresses for the vinegar

Table salt (or sea salt or kosher salt)

Basin, large bowl, or container—to pour the apple cider vinegar into and dip towels in to wring out

Plastic sheet or heavy, large towel (optional)—to place under the limb being treated to protect the sheets

Electric heating pad (optional)—to maintain the heat

Solution of baking soda and water; grain alcohol—to cleanse the area after the pack is removed

FREQUENCY OF APPLICATION

Once or twice a day (as a massage), 1 hour 2 to 3 times daily, daily for 3 weeks, every other day, every 3 to 5 days, 2 to 3 times weekly

LENGTH OF TIME OF APPLICATION

Ten to 15 minutes, 20 minutes, 30 minutes, 1 hour, until condition is relieved, several weeks, 3 to 5 weeks

LOCATION OF APPLICATION

Abdomen, across lumbar, along sciatic nerve, along spine, ankles, areas of acute conditions, areas of distress, between shoulders, elbows, fingernails, feet, hands, hips, knees, joints, painful areas, sternum, wrist

WHEN TO APPLY THE PACK

After abrasions have healed; after removal of bandage, brace, or cast; evenings before retiring; prior to adjustments

SIZE OF PACK

Large enough to cover injured or painful area

EXPECTED EFFECTS/PURPOSES

Produces " . . . a drawing from the glands and from the soft tissue of the body those poisons in the form of a perspiration . . . " (829-1)

Helps knit broken bones and dissolves fluids accumulated at ends of broken bones

Strengthens muscles and bruised tendons; gives better elasticity

Stimulates circulation

Brings " . . . a renewed activity of cartilaginous rebuilding . . . " (33-1)

Relieves tension, strain, pain, soreness, and swelling

Gives strength to the vertebrae

Promotes relaxation

Will " . . . *enliven* the tissue." (4876-1)

Takes away inflammation in cartilage
Supplies nerve energy " . . . to retract, rebuild . . . " (538-10)

DIRECTIONS

Several ways are given for using apple cider vinegar and salt. One way involves applying the vinegar by itself; this can be done for treating a muscle strain or sprain. (In medical terminology a sprain is a sudden twisting or wrenching of a joint, which results in the tearing, stretching, or partial rupture of a ligament. Subsequent damage to blood vessels creates hemorrhaging into the tissue, as well as nerve, muscle, and tendon damage. The area can also become swollen and inflamed. Closely related, a strain is an injury due to excessive tension, force, or overexertion of some part of the musculature, or from a wrenching or twisting that results in undue stretching of muscles or ligaments. Swelling does not occur in a strain.)

To care for either of these conditions, bathe the painful area with the vinegar, then apply a cloth or a towel rung out (not entirely dry) with vinegar and lay it on the skin. After twenty-four hours following the injury, you may add heat to the pack by means of an electric heating pad or a hot salt pack.

Application of heat soothes tired, stiff muscles and achy joints and can speed the healing process. While an electric heating pad may be convenient and useful, salt is also an excellent retainer of heat. The additional weight of salt adds a comforting quality to the treatment.

Directions for making a hot salt pack can be found on the Web site eHow.com, since the treatment is not as frequently used today as in the past. While the readings usually suggest ordinary table salt (sodium chloride, iodized), this Web site recommends the use of kosher or sea salt. Heat about two pounds of salt in a pot over medium heat and stir it with a wooden spoon. Stirring will evenly distribute the heat. After ten minutes, pour the hot salt into a cotton pillowcase or double-bag it with another pillowcase to help hold the salt inside the bag. Twist the ends or tuck them in so that the salt remains in the pillowcase. Next, place the pillowcase either on the painful area or over the vinegar pack. Some readings mention adding vinegar to the salt after it is placed in the pillowcase. When the heat subsides, the salt can be reheated up to five times before it no longer retains the heat.

Another way of utilizing salt, noted in the majority of cases from the readings, combines it with the apple cider vinegar. It can be applied in one of two ways: dampened with the vinegar and rubbed over the painful joint—massaged into the tissue, or sprinkled onto a vinegar-soaked cloth and placed on the affected area. Leave it on as long as you wish or have time for. Afterward, remove the pack and bathe the area with a weak solution of baking soda and water (a teaspoon of baking soda to a cup of warm water), followed by a rub with grain alcohol. This final rub will help close the pores and prevent congestion. (1100–35)

DIRECTIONS FROM THE READINGS

For a female adult suffering with a strained ligament (reading given on September 20, 1927):

> (Q) How long should the massage with the vinegar and salt be kept up?
> (A) For at least three weeks. Each day. If there is severe pain, *heat* same and apply it in a pack. There will be some retractions from the application of these properties if these are massaged well, see? One saturated solution—that is, dissolve all the salt that the quantity will hold, which would be about three to four *tablespoonsful* of the vinegar and near the same quantity of the salt, see? Make this at each time. This may be made sufficient for three to four quantities or two to three days' use at one time. Well that this be *warmed* when applied, but massage well (by the hand) into the limbs. This will remove the soreness and trouble, for this is from strained muscular tissue . . .   4511-2

For a sixty-seven-year-old man with neuritis tendencies (reading given on December 16, 1940):

> . . . apply the heavy salt pack (coarse heavy salt, you see) saturated with Pure Apple Vinegar. This heated and applied will relieve any tension or strain, and the reaction of the sedatives and also the healing

forces, as well as the rubs given as indicated, will continue to keep improvements. Put the salt in a sack or bag, see? then saturate—with the vinegar.   2051-3

Mrs. [5364], a forty–one–year–old woman, suffered from pelvic cellulitis that caused severe back pain for sixteen years (reading given on July 25, 1944):

Should there be periods when there is greater pain, take a single cloth saturated with apple vinegar (this is not to be used until the adjustments have been made, see?). Dip this in vinegar, rinse it out and then cover same and apply to the area aching, and apply salt heat to this. These will relieve the tensions.   5364-1

For a fifty–eight–year–old woman with a sprained ankle (reading given on November 10, 1940):

Each evening, when ready to retire, apply a hot wet bandage about the ankle and the irritated area. Do this for five to ten minutes, to open the pores of the skin thoroughly. Then follow this with a massage using an almost saturated solution of iodized salt and pure apple vinegar; not put on in packs, but massaged gently—not hard, as to break the skin, but do not merely pat it on. Massage it with the fingers, gently, for about twenty minutes; and we will find that this will prove very beneficial. This may then be sponged off, of course, and a *gentle* bandage may be put on if so desired—not tied on, nor as a rubber bandage, but a gentle bandage for the evening. But in a few days we will find great relief from this distress here . . .   805-5

A forty–year–old woman had a fractured leg and was still on crutches; she had been hit by a truck in September 1942 (reading given on January 29, 1944):

We would here add a massage, after each hydrotherapy treatment, for keeping the system purified, using table salt, (preferably iodized) saturated with pure apple vinegar. Don't rub so hard as to break the skin in the joint itself, but so that the body will absorb all that it will. This will help strengthen the tendons and muscles and give better elasticity, as well as aiding the general body.   3608-1

TESTIMONIALS/RESULTS

Mrs. [1100], a forty–seven year old, received her thirty–fifth reading on January 27, 1943. On the first of February, she wrote to Edgar Cayce:

"The reading arrived yesterday and I want to thank you for again helping me when I needed it so badly. These 'catches' in my back were so severe that I could not move or breathe without severe pain. However, since using the salt and vinegar stupes it has just about cleared up entirely. I did not know to sponge off the area with soda water {*baking soda and water*} and alcohol until the reading arrived and have quite a bad case of hives, which I believe is due to absorbing too much vinegar. However, am taking some Milk of Magnesia to neutralize same in system. Anyway, am much better, thanks to Him and to you." 1100-35, Report #1

Dr. Harold Reilly, a physiotherapist who worked closely with Cayce, received a letter dated July 19, 1968, from Mrs. Ann Milano:

"I must also say a word about Cayce remedy 304-3 (Salt and Vinegar massage) of 4/2/23 {*referring to the reading on that date*}, which helped my daughter heal a sprained hand. She was able to move it after an application. This after nothing helped for a year."   304-3, Report #4

Another letter to Edgar Cayce, written on January 17, 1941, by Mrs. [805], contained this short notice:

" . . . I used the vinegar and salt on my ankle with excellent results. It is much better . . . "   805-6, Report #1

No mention is made of what was actually the matter with the ankle.

Cayce in his letters during his waking state often gave physical advice to others. To Mrs. [1866], a fifty–eight–year–old woman who had sprained wrists, he wrote on March 23, 1943:

> "Hope your wrists are coming along all right. When you take off the casts, be sure to massage the wrists with salt saturated with pure apple vinegar, and they will not give you any further trouble—as such sprains do sometimes when weather is to be bad . . . "   1866-11, Report #2

ADDITIONAL INFORMATION

Vinegar is perhaps the oldest healing home remedy. An early Assyrian medical text describes an application of vinegar to treat ear pain. In biblical times it was used to dress wounds and infectious sores. During the U.S. Civil War, vinegar was credited with saving the lives of thousands of soldiers, as it was applied routinely as a disinfectant on wounds.

Essentially vinegar is spoiled wine, most likely accidentally discovered about ten thousand years ago around the time wine was discovered. Its word origin may be French: *vinaigre* (*vin*—wine; *aigre*—sour). Technically it is an acidic liquid made from almost any mildly sweet or alcoholic beverage such as wine, cider, or beer, though health benefits are usually linked to vinegar made from apple cider.

In times past the elaborate process of souring apple cider into vinegar often had magical overtones. However, a tiny microorganism, the vinegar bacillus, produces what is known as an "acetous fermentation," creating water and acetic acid, which gives vinegar its characteristic tart taste. Two separate and distinct fermentation processes are required to make vinegar. In the first, sugar is changed to alcohol, and in the second, alcohol is changed to acetic acid. This process was thought to confer a special healing ability on the end product, hence its reported traditional use as an enduring health remedy.

OTHER USES FOR APPLE CIDER VINEGAR

In contrast to vinegar's frequent use as a spice for salads, a weight-loss aid, and an alkalizer for the body, nearly fifty readings caution against ingesting it in one's diet. Yet enthusiasts claim a long list of ailments that reportedly can be cured or prevented by taking apple cider vinegar internally. Consistently the Cayce readings advise individuals not to put vinegar on raw salads or to eat any food seasoned or canned with vinegar, thus avoiding highly seasoned foods or foods treated with vinegar such as pickles and pickled beets or carrots. " . . . For the basis of such acid is not good in the body–structural forces . . . " (2514-14)

With some individuals, vinegar was irritating to the digestion or would produce an over acidity in the stomach. The majority of the dietary excerpts, however, simply state to avoid it, with no specific reason given. " . . . Never any preparations, as salads, carrying vinegar—unless wine vinegar is used," one individual was told. (2991-2) Of course, a number of these people had health problems that conceivably could be exacerbated by ingesting vinegar.

Indirectly, the readings mention that vinegar has a beneficial effect in hair rinses that contain it as an ingredient. The comment was made during a series of queries on Furfluf, a fur cleanser that Mrs. [1000] was trying to manufacture and market, in which Cayce simply acknowledged vinegar's good effects in a hair rinse. (1000-19)

One fifty–one–year–old woman asked what " . . . special combination {could} be used to prevent serious results from sunburn." The answer in reading 601-22 was: "There is no better than plain, pure apple vinegar!" Sunburn is an inflamed skin condition caused by prolonged exposure to the sun's ultraviolet rays. The affected area becomes red, hot, and tender, and in severe cases blisters may form. Avoiding any outdoor activity in the middle of the day is frequently noted, roughly from 11:00 a.m. to 2:00 p.m., since during that time period the sun " . . . carries too *great* a quantity of the actinic rays that make for destructive forces to the superficial circulation . . . " (934-2) Actinic rays are light rays (in particular, the violet and ultraviolet parts of the spectrum) that produce chemical changes. So while beneficial results may be derived from absorption of the sun's ultraviolet rays [giving " . . . strength and vitality to the nerves and muscular forces . . . " (3172-2)], caution and warnings need to be heeded, guarding against overexposure.

No mention is made in the readings of the actual technique for applying the vinegar to the sunburned area, but soaking a washcloth in the vinegar and laying it against the skin or patting the vinegar onto the skin is noted in some home remedy texts.

As an addition to bathwater, vinegar and salt were suggested in the following excerpt: " . . . bathe the hips and {pubis} with water containing vinegar and salt, not too strong but just enough to strengthen the body from the over strained condition of the system {vulvitis} . . . " (4449–1)

See also under the heading *Other Uses for Coffee Grounds* in the chapter "Coffee Foot Bath" for using vinegar, olive oil, and re-steamed coffee grounds as a tanning formula for the skin.

Considering its many uses, apple cider vinegar remains a stable substance and a permanent fixture in one's kitchen cabinet.

Apple Diet

The term *diet*, as used in the Cayce readings, most often does not mean what is ordinarily thought of: a weight-loss regimen. More likely *diet* refers to a way to detoxify one's body, to cleanse the system, and to achieve a healthier balance. The apple diet is one of several mentioned in the readings (grapes, bananas, and citrus fruit are other examples). This mono-diet is most familiar to individuals as well as the one most often recommended. It involves eating only raw apples for three days, followed by a dose of olive oil (*see also* the chapter on "Olive Oil").

In *The Edgar Cayce Handbook for Health Through Drugless Therapy*, author Dr. Harold Reilly states: "Since most people are toxic to a greater or lesser degree, I have found that a good cleansing routine with the apple-diet regimen is the first step toward improving assimilation and elimination for anyone. If one is reasonably well, the detoxification will bring about an almost euphoric feeling of well-being and provide inexpensive and effective insurance against disease. If one is not well, the apple-cleansing regimen is an excellent beginning of a therapeutic program." (p. 221)

INDICATIONS

Acidity, adhesions, anemia, arthritis, bronchitis, cerebral hemorrhage, childbirth (aftereffects), constipation, debilitation, epilepsy, headaches, hypertension, incoordination of nervous system, intestinal worms, menopause, neurasthenia, neuritis tendencies, pelvic disorders, pin-worms, poor assimilations, poor eliminations, spinal subluxations, stroke, toxemia

CONTRAINDICATIONS

Check with a physician before embarking on any such type of diet; not recommended for everyone, as some people develop headaches, cramps, or other symptoms because they cannot handle the apples; follow the instructions carefully—three days of raw apples only, fol-lowed by a dose of olive oil; if you have a history of liver or gallbladder problems, take a minimum amount of olive oil; do not use castor oil packs while on the diet: "*Do not* attempt to use the Apple Diet as a cleanser, if using the {*Castor*} Oil Packs . . . But do not mix the two courses; either follow the one or the other!" (543-27)

MATERIALS NEEDED

Enough organic apples to eat over a 3–day period [for example, first day: 6 to 8 apples, second day: 4 to 6 apples, third day: 2 to 4 apples (some people may eat 8 to 10 apples each day; others as few as only 1 a day)]—jenneting variety: that is, Delicious, Oregon Red, Arkansas Black, Russet, Sheep Nose, or Jonathan; not the Winesap (see also *Testimonials/ Results* and *Additional Information*)

Bottle of pure, extra virgin olive oil—to take after the diet is com-pleted

FREQUENCY OF APPLICATION

Three days of eating raw apples only; coffee, if desired, may be drunk, but without cream, milk, and/or sugar in it; lots of water (suggested: 6 to 8 glasses daily) should also be drunk during the treatment

AMOUNT OF DOSAGE

(Apples) As many as you want to consume in three days

(Olive oil) At the end of the third day in the evening before retiring: two to three teaspoons, one or two tablespoons, half a teacup, half a glass, half a cup—removes old fecal matter, cleanses the system of impurities, prevents inclination of gas formation, and changes the activity through the whole alimentary canal

WHEN TO TAKE THE APPLE DIET

After a series of castor oil packs; when the system needs clearing or cleansing

LENGTH OF TIME OF APPLICATION

May need to be repeated to be truly effective, next month, once a month for two or three months, every three months

EXPECTED EFFECTS/PURPOSES

Purifies the body system

Cleanses the activities of the liver and kidneys and " . . . all toxic forces from any system . . . " (820-2)

Is a good eliminant for the body

Gets " . . . rid of the tendencies for neuritic conditions in the joints of the body . . . " (1409-9)

Increases eliminations and cleanses the alimentary canal

DIRECTIONS

According to the readings, raw apples are only to be consumed alone, *with no other food;* however, baked, cooked, or roasted apples are acceptable *with other foods.* Reading 935-1 states: " . . . Apples should only be eaten when cooked; preferably roasted and with butter or hard sauce on same, with cinnamon and spice." Why is this?

Simone Gabbay, nutritionist and columnist for *Venture Inward* magazine, says it's difficult to speculate; perhaps "because the raw apple has such a powerful cleansing effect on the body, it could interfere with the normal process of assimilation of nutrients from other foods." (*Nourish-*

ing the Body Temple, pp. 85–86) Elsewhere, the readings describe raw apples
" . . . taken alone as a diet for the eliminations . . . " (1206–8)

On December 12, 1926, a fifty-four-year-old woman asked: "Why are
apples not good?" The response was:

> In this particular condition, and any condition of this nature {*general
> debilitation, nervous tension, assimilation/elimination incoordina-
> tion*}, the apple produces an acid that produces portion of the bitter-
> ness in the system, by the action of regurgitation in the duodenum
> {*first section of small intestine*}, produced by the excretions from the
> pancreas being overcharged by this nature of apples in the system. We
> have given the reason.   325-14

The strong, cleansing effect of this three-day apple diet is achieved in
a fairly straightforward way. Eat as many apples—preferably organic—
as you want or need for the three days. If the apples are not organic,
they should be peeled. Cayce also stated: " . . . Beware of apples, unless
of the jenneting variety . . . " (509–2) (See also *Testimonials/Results* and
Additional Information.) Drink plenty of water during that time and coffee,
if you wish, but without milk, cream, and/or sugar. While you may stay
active during the time of this diet, you should not overtire or strain
yourself with strenuous activities.

On the evening of the third day, just before going to bed, take a dose
of pure olive oil. Amounts in the readings range from two to three
teaspoons to half a teacup, or half a glass. If you have a liver condition
or gallbladder problems, drink only the minimum amount of olive oil.
This is a one-time consumption of the oil.

When you begin to eat again on the fourth day, don't " . . . overgorge
the system . . . " (1850–3); eat regularly and normally, but do not choose
foods that are too rich or highly seasoned. Some individuals were advised to repeat the three-day diet monthly for two or three months, in
order for it to be effective. Dr. Harold Reilly recommends taking colonics
during the three days, particularly on the first day, or an enema at the
end of the first or second day. If possible, get another colonic or enema

in the evening of the third day. These hydrotherapy treatments may help prevent headaches, cramps, or other discomforts that the diet may produce when individuals are detoxifying; otherwise, one may begin to reabsorb the toxins being thrown off from the lower colon. Dr. Reilly also suggests taking a fume or steam bath (unless contraindicated), having a massage, and doing some general exercise during the three days.

DIRECTIONS FROM THE READINGS
For a twenty-nine-year-old woman with epilepsy (reading given on December 15, 1937):

> For this, then, as we find, occasionally—not too often—take the periods for the cleansing of the system with the use of the *apple diet;* that is:
> At least for three days—two days or three days—take *nothing* except *apples—raw apples!* Of course, coffee may be taken if so desired, but no other foods but the raw apples. And then after the last meal of apples on the third day, or upon retiring on that evening following the last meal of apples, drink half a cup of Olive Oil.
> This will tend to cleanse the system.
> Raw apples otherwise taken (except at such cleansing periods) are not so well for the body . . .   543-26

For a fifty-nine-year-old woman with debilitation and neuritis, stiffness on the left side of her face, and a swollen stomach (reading given on October 19, 1937):

> . . . the regular Apple Diet would be *well* for the body—*but don't try to work like a horse when you are on the apple diet!* or else we will find it will be more detrimental than helpful! But these cleansings will prevent the accumulations of gas, the pressures that make for the neuritis through the portions of the body. But just be consistent.   307-14

For a twenty-four-year-old woman with nervous system incoordination, spinal subluxations, and poor eliminations (reading given on February 21, 1944):

Here, one good eliminant for this body would be to go on the apple diet—at least every three months; that is, eat nothing for three days except raw apples, preferably the Jonathan variety or a kindred variety. Follow this with at least two to three teaspoonful of Olive Oil; that is, after the three days. This is to change the activity through the whole alimentary canal.   3673-1

TESTIMONIALS/RESULTS

Mrs. [639], who received her second reading from Cayce on August 21, 1934, when she was sixty-three years old, wrote a letter to Cayce dated March 21, 1935:

" . . . in your March 1935 *Bulletin* {*former A.R.E. publication*} under 'Health Hints' {*regarding the apple diet*} . . . Will you kindly advise me what the Jenneting variety apples are, where they grow, and where they can be purchased . . . "   639-2, Report #6

(See also *Additional Information.*)

On April 23, 1935, Edgar Cayce wrote that he had made some inquiries and thought it was the same variety as Delicious, Arkansas Black, and the Russet: " . . . and there is one, of course, called the original Jenneting. Haven't tried this out myself as yet but as I usually do am going to try it, for would never want to be the means of giving something for someone that I wouldn't try myself." (639-2, Report #6)

She later reported on her experiences on April 19, 1936:

"I have been taking the apple diet once a month for three months; I think it a splendid thing and I get along with it very well with the exception that the olive oil makes me so sick at my stomach. I am wondering how it would do to take it {*the apple diet*} every two weeks for one day and a half with ¼ glass of oil? Maybe that amount of oil wouldn't affect me so badly. Mr. [550] took it the last time I did but the oil didn't make him sick. I believe you wrote once that you had taken the diet for half the time prescribed and would like to ask if you used half the amount of oil in doing so."   639-2, Report #11

On May 6, 1936, Edgar Cayce replied:

"Perhaps you take too much of the olive oil with your apple diet. I only took half a teacup—that, it seems to me, is less than the glass, isn't it? Have found excellent results with only a day of the diet, and decreasing the oil according to the days taken. Try that and see if you do not have good results."   639-2, Report #12

In one instance, in a reading on himself, Cayce received this information: "Too much picric acid has been a part of the diet here." (294-194) Gladys Davis made this notation: "I think EC had been on an apple diet for a day; had to stop, he was suffering so." This reading on September 29, 1939, was given several years after the above correspondence.

ADDITIONAL INFORMATION

Apples are a good source of vitamins and minerals: A, C, B complex, calcium, potassium, phosphorus, and magnesium. They contain pectin, a fiber which has a gentle laxative effect, and are also high in bioflavonoids (antioxidant compounds).

Water and coffee (one reading, 1597-2, mentioned the choice of " . . . a cereal drink . . . ") were the only food items that might be consumed with the raw apple diet; not to be consumed: milk, bread, and yeast were specifically noted.

. . . Raw apples are not well {*for the three-day apple diet*} unless they are of the jenneting variety . . .   820-2

. . . The jenneting or Jonathan variety is better than those of the woody stock; as the Winesap.   257-167

"Jenneting," according to one dictionary of obsolete words, is an early pear resembling the jenneting apple, so named because it ripens on St. John's day, June 24. *Webster's New Twentieth Century Dictionary* defines it as "a species of early apples."

Other varieties of apples suggested in the readings include Arkansas Black, Sheep Nose, Delicious, Oregon Red, and Jonathan. The Delicious (the yellow and red) might be the easiest to locate in grocery stores. Some people prefer the yellow variety, which contains the most pectin (noted by Dr. Reilly), a substance which helps reduce cholesterol.

Though the three-day apple diet is intended in the readings as a purifying and cleansing diet rather than a means of losing weight, weight loss may be a natural result of decreasing food intake while on the diet.

Atomidine

Although mentioned in the Cayce readings over 2,500 times as Atomidine (pronounced *ah-TOM-uh-deen*), this highly useful product, discovered in 1914, was originally sold under the name Beslin (as well as other designations) and distributed by Schieffelin and Company in New York City until the early 1940s. At that time the two-ounce bottle of liquid sold for $1.00. Now it is available under the label Atomic Iodine™, a description, according to the readings, of just what Atomidine is.

From the multiple uses to which the readings refer, it can appear to be a "wonder drug." Diluted internal uses include it as a mouth and gum wash, as a nasal and throat spray or gargle, as a solution in enemas, as a douche, and most often taken in small doses in a glass of water for glandular and iodine deficiencies. Used externally, it can be applied as a local antiseptic, a steam bath additive, a pack, a massage lubricant, a stupe, and as a solution for the Radio-Active Appliance.

Almost always, Atomidine is used in conjunction with other treatments. Its value lies in that it is iodine in a form that is apparently less toxic to the body than what is available from other commercial sources. Though probably safe for *external* use by most anyone, it should be used with great care when ingested *internally*. Its high iodine content can be harmful to some who might take too large a dosage, while others could be sensitive to even minute amounts. Each drop of the solution contains approximately 1/100 grain of iodine, supplying about six times the minimum daily requirement of iodine; "legally (it) is a prescription item when used internally," and should be taken only under a physician's care (*An Edgar Cayce Home Medicine Guide*, p. 5).

INDICATIONS
(Internal) Arthritis, asthma, baldness, cysts (on womb), dizziness, excessive hair, glandular disorders, goiter, hypertension, infantile paralysis, leukemia, neuritis, nodules, poison ivy, scaly or tough skin, skin eruptions, sluggish thyroid, split fingernails, swollen joints, tooth decay, vertigo

(Douche) Feminine hygiene, infection, inflammation

(Oral—mouth and gum wash) Acidity; (nasal, throat spray, gargle) Cold prevention, sinus irritations, sore throat

(External) Bites, boils, cuts, dental problems, hangnails, hard nails, infantile paralysis, ingrown toenails, mouth sores, poison ivy, rashes, venereal disease

(Fume bath) Insomnia, tumors

(Massage lubricant, diluted) Neck carbuncles, stiff muscles, swollen glands

(Pack) Menstruation problems, swollen joints

(Radio-Active Appliance) Solution—for purifying, inflammation

(Stupe) Liver and stomach pain, soreness, stiff limbs, swelling

CONTRAINDICATIONS
Take internally only under a doctor's supervision; may overstimulate thyroid gland, causing nervousness, irritability, skin rashes, insomnia, increased heart rate; do not take with other iodine–containing drugs such as thyroid pills, heart stimulants (2366-7), multiple vitamin or mineral tablets containing iodine, or if you are already obtaining iodine in your diet (by frequently eating seafood) from Calcios, Calcidin, or

Codiron (1206-9), from certain formulas (such as Herbal Tonic 636) or sea air; do not use when beginning the use of the Radio-Active Appliance (2514-1); not at same time period as diathermy (905-1); not with Valentine's Extract of Liver or Ventriculin with Iron (1173-1); not on the same days as alcohol, yeast (908-5), cod-liver oil, KalDak (nutritional supplement, no longer available, 3445-1), kelp salt, Epsom salt baths, or electrotherapy [infrared (275-29, 808-5), Violet Ray]; some individuals were told not to have spinal manipulations on the days of taking Atomidine, while others were told it was acceptable

MATERIALS NEEDED
Bottle of Atomidine
Cloth or towel—if using Atomidine with pack or stupe

FREQUENCY OF APPLICATION
(Internal) Once or twice a day, usually a rest period, then repeat cycle (cf. individual readings for wide variety of frequencies and amounts)
(Douche) Occasionally, once a day, every other day, once a week, once a month
(Enema) Twice a week
(Gargle) Twice a day, once to twice a week
(Massage) Every week
(Pack) 20 to 30 minutes, 1 hour, all day
(Spray) Once a day or every 2 days, occasionally, in evening before retiring, 2 to 3 times a week

AMOUNT OF DOSAGE
(Internal—in a survey of over 300 readings there were 75 different ways to take Atomidine; use only under a doctor's supervision)—*Ratio of Atomidine to amount of water* (small sample): 1 drop in ½ glass water for 5 days, leave off 5 days, repeat; 1 drop twice a day; 1 drop first day, 2 drops second day, 3 drops third day; 6 to 8 drops: whole glass of water
(Douche) 1 teaspoon: 1 or 1½ quarts water; 1 tablespoon: 2 quarts water
(Enema) 1 teaspoon: 1 pint water, then place in quart of water con-

taining baking soda and salt (935-2)

(External) 1 teaspoon: ½ glass water

(Gargle) Weakened solution; 5 or 30 to 40 drops: ½ glass water; 1 teaspoon: ⅓ glass water; 1 teaspoon: 2 ounces distilled water; 2 teaspoons: ½ glass water

(Massage) 10 drops: 2 ounces distilled water; a few drops: 1 tablespoon water; ½ Atomidine: ½ distilled water

(Radio-Active Appliance) One-half commercial strength: ½ distilled water

(Spray) Weakened solution; 30% solution Atomidine; 1 teaspoon: 1 ounce distilled water; 1 teaspoon: 2 ounces distilled water; 1 part Atomidine: 10 parts distilled (not tap) water; 1 drop: 10 drops water; 2 teaspoons: ½ glass water

(Stupe) 1 tablespoon: 1 quart water

WHEN TO TAKE THE ATOMIDINE

(Internal) Mornings; before morning meal and before retiring; ½ to ¾ hour before morning meal and three or four or five o'clock in afternoon; before, after, or during the period of taking Epsom salt bath; when the spittle and urine are acidic; when hydrotherapy treatments, including colonics, are taken

(Douche) After or before menstrual period

(Gargle and mouth rinse) After brushing the teeth

LENGTH OF TIME OF APPLICATION

(Internal) Three days; for 5, 6, 7, or 8 days; 10 days, rest for 5 days, then repeat; 30 to 60 days; several months; 2 or 3 months; repeat cycle 3 times; one week rest, then repeat cycle; two series; one week a month; throughout the year; until relief is obtained

(Pack) Five days

EXPECTED EFFECTS/PURPOSES

Purifies and cleanses the glands and stimulates thyroid

Creates a " . . . perfect coordination between the glandular forces of the body . . . " (1933-1)

Builds " . . . strength to the whole anatomical condition of the body . . . " (1475-1)

Helps to tone and maintain a more equal balance in the system—if "*used* properly!" (358-1)

Strengthens the nails of the fingers and toes

Stimulates circulation through the lungs, heart, liver, and kidneys

DIRECTIONS

Because the dosages and cycles for taking Atomidine orally vary so much, it is highly recommended to study the Circulating File on one's particular health condition to determine the proper amount to consume. Since a number of variations might be offered, choose an individual of the same sex whose physical condition and age closely match yours, then follow the suggestions in that reading. Read also the Circulating File on "Atomidine" to gain a better understanding of its many uses. Additionally, check and work with your personal physician as to the proper course to follow.

Overstimulation to the thyroid gland, which traps iodine and processes it into thyroid hormones, can result in nervousness, irritability, skin rashes, insomnia, or an increase in heart rate. It should *not* be taken with other iodine-containing drugs such as thyroid pills, heart stimulants (2366-7), any multiple vitamin or mineral tablet containing iodine, or if you are already obtaining iodine in your diet (e.g.: seafood), from Calcios, Codiron (1206-9), Calcidin, or from certain formulas (such as Herbal Tonic 636).

Despite these cautions on internal applications, the readings state: " . . . This will not only be a curative property, but a *preventative* . . . especially for any form of disorder in glands *or* tissue of body." (358-2). Reiterated throughout this body of information is its purpose, when taken orally, as a gland purifier and cleanser, especially affecting the thyroid, thymus, adrenals, and other ductless glands. Another reading states that " . . . most glands function as machinery would under oil. The iodine being the oil for the gland, see?" (294-130)

DIRECTIONS FROM THE READINGS

For a fifty-year-old accountant complaining of calluses on the feet who desired to improve his glandular function (reading given on August 1, 1935):

> As indicated, it is not necessary for the Atomidine to be *continually* taken, but when there are the influences necessary for the secretions or the activities of the glands (with which the Atomidine functions so well), it is well to have same on hand and to take a few drops for two, three, four or five days. Then discontinue until there is seen the necessity for adding same to make for the activity of the glands, to make for the hormones in the blood supply to keep the proper balance and necessary coordination in the system.   270-34

An adult woman (no age given) had pelvic disorders resulting in vaginal discharges (reading given on May 12, 1941):

> At least every day, until the irritation and discharge is better, *do* have the Atomidine douche—body-temperature. The proportions would be a teaspoonful of Atomidine to each quart of water, used—having the water body temperature. Then after the Atomidine douche, use a warm douche with Glyco-Thymoline in same—about a tablespoonful to the quart of water. The Atomidine is the acid and the Glyco-Thymoline the alkalin{*e*}, you see. The Atomidine douche is destructive to the tissue that has become irritated or sore; while the Glyco-Thymoline douche following same is an antiseptic. Both are antiseptic in their natures, but one is an acid while the other is an alkaline. Have these at the same time, but take the Atomidine douche first each day; preferably when ready to retire.   654-9

A forty-four-year-old male, suffering from an acidic condition, with tendencies toward neuritis, hemorrhoids, and baldness (reading given on May 29, 1943):

> Use a very weak solution of the Atomidine as a massage for the hair. To

two ounces of Distilled Water put ten drops of the Atomidine. Use this on the head and hair. Put this on dry—that is, with the hair dry. *Then* use the soap, and preferably tar soap afterward, as the shampoo—for the thorough cleansing of same. Do this, and we will find better conditions for this body.   1727-2

For a twenty-nine-year-old woman with pyorrhea tendencies and nervous system and glandular incoordinations (reading given on January 16, 1937):

(Q) Is there any special precaution one can take to keep from getting the "flu"?
(A) Spraying the nasal passages and throat occasionally with a thirty percent solution of Atomidine—that is, commercial strength—will most insure not getting same; provided the body is kept alkaline with the diets.   808-5

For a fifty-six-year-old medical doctor with anemia and poor assimilations who was cured of a throat hemorrhage (reading given on February 2, 1938):

Use the Atomidine spray preferably of an evening before retiring. The proportions would be a teaspoonful of the Atomidine (commercial strength) to an ounce of Distilled Water (not tap water, but distilled water). Use as a nasal spray and as a throat spray. Use preferably in an atomizer of hard rubber, or be very careful that any *metal* parts to the one used are thoroughly cleansed after each usage of same—or before it is used again *sterilize same!* and do not let the metal parts (if such is used) remain in that portion of the Atomidine Solution not used! But do not use a metal spray for the Atomidine spray solution, if at all practical.   1210-4

For a forty-three-year-old man who had had multiple sclerosis for fourteen months (reading given on October 7, 1943):

Every day, where there is swelling in joints and in portions of the body, dampen a cloth with Atomidine (full strength), and wrap it about that area. Leave this on for an hour or until the cloth is entirely dried out from the absorption. Keep this up for five days.   3270-1

A forty–two–year–old man who later stated that his main problem was homosexuality used the Wet–Cell Appliance along with taking Atomidine (reading given on November 15, 1943):

First we would begin taking internally small quantities of Atomidine, to produce excess iodine in the body. Take one drop in half a glass of water each morning before breakfast for five days.   3364-1

TESTIMONIALS/RESULTS

A follow–up letter written by Miss [954] to Edgar Cayce on February 8, 1938, reported on the progress of [1210], a fifty–six–year–old MD who had experienced a throat hemorrhage (see *Directions from the Readings*). She wrote:

"Just a note to tell you that there is a distinct pick-up in the Doctor's vitality . . . much better coordinated in his thinking as if relieved of toxins. I think it most important that the sprays were given, for he tells me that although the Atomidine spray was distinctly painful at first . . . it is no longer. It is quite evident that the reading did discover an unguessed spot of infection."   1210-4, Report #1

Mr. [1467], who was twenty–eight years old when he received his seventeenth reading on March 12, 1943, was given this recommendation:

Even with the trouble with the finger, it will be found that the application of Atomidine *in* the body and *to* the body is beneficial, for these are the activities within the body that aid in purifying glands, thus acting much in the same manner as releasing by manipulative forces a pressure where congestion may be caused.   1467-17

Years later on July 8, 1966, he reported that the past fall he had suffered with arthritis in his lower back, being immobilized for two to three months. He remembered about the Atomidine [in his reading] and began taking it, watching his diet, and the arthritis started getting better. He was now entirely free of it.

The next two accounts are from a report that Edgar Cayce sent to Dr. S.A. Bisey, the discoverer of Atomidine, on February 28, 1933, describing some individuals' successes with using his product.

> "{*The*} case of Miss [951] from ... Ohio—eighteen years of age {*who had a total of seven readings*}; had been suffering for several years with what had been diagnosed as arthritis. Physicians had despaired of anything being done, to prevent continual hardening and enlarging of joints, and stiffness arising from such. There was gradual contraction of tendons and muscles from all joints, especially hands and feet.
>
> "A course of Atomidine was prescribed {*first reading given on October 21, 1932*}, small dosage three times a day for a period of three weeks; then a rest period of a week, then another three weeks of the Atomidine with baths and other recommendations, including strict diet.
>
> "At the end of four weeks the patient was free entirely of any suffering, soreness, stiffness, and to date—now nearly six months—no return of any bad symptoms.
>
> "The treatment is still being continued, with a reduced quantity of Atomidine."   1734-5, Report #11

Mrs. [272] from Alabama was thirty-two years old at the time of her first reading on October 29, 1930, and had a total of nine readings.

> "{*She*} had a very bad case of infection from G.C. {*gonococcal; gonorrhea*} germs, which had been disturbing her for some months. Treatments from physicians had failed to clear the bloodstream or to give any relief from local infections.
>
> "Atomidine was prescribed in courses, 8 to 10 drops twice a day, and douches carrying Atomidine also.

"Almost immediately there was noted relief from the eruptions, as well as from the severe pains that had continued for some time.

"The condition has cleared entirely, and the body attributes her relief to the use of Atomidine—which cleansed her body of the dreaded condition."   1734-5, Report #11

ADDITIONAL INFORMATION

On March 7, 1933, Dr. Sunkar (also spelled Sunker) A. Bisey, a distinguished Hindu scientist and inventor (called the "Edison of India") who discovered Atomidine and several years earlier requested readings on its proper manufacture and marketing, sent a flier to Cayce which offered this information:

" . . . Atomidine is a stable compound of iodine in a saline solution that liberates the element in an atomic or nascent state on contact with an excess of solvent, such as the fluids of the body . . . By liberating nascent or atomic iodine, Atomidine furnishes the organism with this element in such a form that it may be readily utilized . . .

"Atomidine acts beneficially in iodine deficiency diseases, gastrointestinal disorders, and asthenic conditions. It has the property of reducing blood-pressure in cases of hypertension. Atomidine is an efficient diuretic and urinary antiseptic, acting in either an acid or alkaline medium."   1734-5, Report #12

Another comment on the proper use of Atomidine comes from reading 1100-8:

(Q) Should the body continue taking the Atomidine internally?
(A) The small portions, yes. This has been indicated, and the use of same as a spray is helpful also.

Take periods of Atomidine; not continued every day but for a week every day, rest a week and begin again. These are more effective than continued, for *any* property. For this may be said to be the manner in which any outside influence acts upon not only this body but any body:

To continue the use of any *one* influence that is active upon the body *continually* is to cause those portions of the system that *produce* same to lose their activity or their significance, and depend upon the supply from without.

But to give stimulation to the system and then refrain from same tends to produce *in* the body that necessary reaction in the glandular system and in the functioning of organs. For the body (normal) produces within itself the necessary elements for its continual reproduction of itself at *all* times. 1100-8

Becoming familiar with your body's physical needs and taking note of various recommendations from the readings for Atomidine will help you make a wise choice for your own particular benefit.

Beef Juice

Beef juice, according to the readings, belongs to the categories of "body-building" and "blood-building" foods. More than 400 readings mention it as a supplement or tonic for stimulating and strengthening the body and to be " . . . taken regularly as medicine . . . " (5374-1) Not to be confused with beef extract, broth, stew, bouillon, or soup, beef juice is a specially prepared food item, to be ingested in small quantities either occasionally or on a regular basis. The juice is extracted from the meat through the process of heat.

INDICATIONS

Aftereffects of surgery, anemia, body strengthening, calcium deficiency, cancer, debilitation, epilepsy, fatigue, flu-like symptoms, glandular disturbance, incoordination: assimilations and eliminations, low stamina, multiple sclerosis, tuberculosis, tumors, weakness; building up resistance, gaining weight

MATERIALS NEEDED

One-quarter pound to ½ pound, or 1 to 1½ pounds of lean round steak or good lean beef

Knife—to cut meat into half-inch cubes and to remove fat
Glass jar or container (with cover)
Boiler or pan—to fill with water and in which to place glass jar
Cloth or wire rack—to place under glass jar in pan
Small container—to refrigerate the juice
Tongs (optional)—to extract the beef cubes after boiling
Cheesecloth (optional)—to strain fat globules after cooking
Patapar paper (optional)—to wrap beef cubes rather than using a
covered glass jar

FREQUENCY OF DOSAGE

(Daily) Ranges from 2 to 6 times; every 15, 20, or 30 minutes; every ½
hour to 1 hour; every 2 to 3 hours; every few hours; every 8 hours; daily
for 2 to 3 weeks, 2 to 3 times in the morning and 2 to 3 times in the
evening; often

(Weekly) Two to 3 times a week

Take " . . . according to the feelings of the body . . . " (1667-1) or as
often " . . . as the appetite calls for same." (538-42)

AMOUNT OF DOSAGE

Small amounts—sipped slowly, not gulped down—taken each time
(amounts, due to individual differences, varied): ½ to ¾ teaspoon; 1 or 2
teaspoons; a few teaspoons; 1 or 2 tablespoons; a few drops or sips; *total
amount per day:* 1 to 3 tablespoons; 1 to 1½ ounces; 4 to 6 ounces; *time it
should take to consume each dosage:* 1 to 1½ minutes; 2, 3, 4, or 5 minutes; at
least 2 or 3 minutes; 10 to 20 minutes; for ½ teaspoon take it in three sips

WHEN TO TAKE THE BEEF JUICE

At each meal (breakfast, lunch, and/or dinner), as an appetizer twenty
to thirty minutes before evening meal, before or after meals, between
meals, after resting a few minutes when returning home from work,
mornings and afternoons, before retiring at bedtime, during the day

EXPECTED EFFECTS/PURPOSES

Produces gastric flow through the intestinal system

Supplies " . . . the necessary proteins and calories for the body . . . " (4330-1)

Strengthens the body

Assists in building " . . . muscle, tissue, bone and structural forces of the body." (142-4)

Relaxes and replenishes the body

Carries vitamins that strengthen the body (noted, in particular, was B-1); also contains iron

DIRECTIONS

Use about one-quarter of a pound to a pound-and-a-half of lean round steak, " . . . diced about half an inch, no fat . . . " (1419-2); " . . . no portions other than that which is of the muscle or tendon . . . no . . . skin portions . . . " (1343-2) " . . . Preferably use the beef from the neck of the animal." (975-5) " . . . or the rump. This is the type of meat to be used to make the juice. More strength will be found in same." (1899-1)

The amount of raw beef would depend upon how long and how often you intend to take the juice. " . . . There will be enough in a pound {of beef} to last for two or three days . . . " (461-1)

After you cut the meat in small chunks [" . . . about the size of a good sized marble or the thumb . . . " (461-1)], being careful to cut away all the fat, place the raw pieces—no water added, in order to make it a *pure* beef juice—in a glass jar that can be covered. Put the jar into a boiler or other stove-top container that is deep enough so that the water added to the pot will cover about one-half to three-fourths of the side of the jar. Cover the top of the jar, but do not seal it tightly. Set the jar on a cloth or a rack placed on the bottom of the pan to prevent the jar from cracking. Then boil the water for about two to four hours. (Option: You may instead place the meat in Patapar paper, tie a bowknot at the top, set the bag in water, and boil the meat. This will preserve the juice.)

The beef juice will build up and accumulate inside the jar during the boiling process. The juice is ready when no trace of pink remains in the juice itself when held to the light and the color is a rich brown. " . . . cook it *done*, the meat, you see . . . then strain off, but don't eat the meat—it isn't good for a dog even! . . . " (418-4) While straining off the juice (may be done with cheesecloth), you can also press the beef cubes or squeeze with tongs to extract any remaining fluid. Remove all traces of fat or tallow, which will solidify on top of the juice. Store the juice in a small container in the refrigerator or other cool place and toss out the worthless meat.

The juice should " . . . be prepared {fresh} every three or four days . . . " (855-1); one reading says, " . . . never {keep it} longer than three days . . . " (1343-2); another advises, " . . . do not keep the same quantity—even in the ice box—over two days, but make fresh . . . " (1658-1), while another says to make a fresh quantity " . . . At least every other day . . . " (2075-1) Several readings (for example, 667-8, 1419-2, 1509-1, 2642-1, and 2978-1) state that it should be made fresh *each day*. Beef juice should never be frozen in order to reuse it.

Take small sips several times daily (see *Frequency of Dosage, Amount of Dosage,* and *When to Take the Beef Juice*). It may be warmed or kept cool (often no temperature suggestion was offered). To suit one's own taste or to tolerate it, a little salt may be added or it may be diluted with water that has been previously boiled (the ratio: one teaspoon water to one tablespoon beef juice).

After sipping the suggested amount, a half ounce to two ounces of red wine by itself or with brown bread or whole wheat crackers may be taken, or simply whole wheat bread or Rye-Krisp or Graham crackers, " . . . which carry little of the starches and sufficient of weight and cleansing for the system itself." (528-3) These additions " . . . make it more palatable." (1343-2) " . . . The beef juice may be sipped or eaten with a whole wheat cracker, and settled or 'chased' (as some might term it) with the wine [an ounce of light wine; this not too sweet, but not the sour wine]." (3123-1) Citrus fruit juices or simply fruit, " . . . as peaches, pineapples and such fruit, or that ordinarily found in a fruit salad . . . " (307-5) may also be taken after sipping the juice.

DIRECTIONS FROM THE READINGS

For an adult male suffering from anemia (reading given on November 28, 1933):

(Q) How should the beef juices be prepared?

(A) Take a pound to a pound and a half of beef—*lean* beef, no fat! Dice it into small pieces . . . Put in a glass jar. Seal the jar, no water in same. Put this in water, with a cloth or something in to prevent from breaking or cracking the jar. Let it boil for two to three hours. Extract the juice. Throw the meat away. Season the juice and take it as directed {*at least one tablespoon each evening before retiring*} . . . Keep in a cool place. Not beef broth, but beef *juice!*   461-1

For a twenty–seven–year–old woman suffering from tuberculosis of the lungs (reading given on April 26, 1943):

Beef juice (though never the meat itself) should be taken rather as medicine, so it will assimilate. This should be prepared fresh at least every day, and a quarter to half a pound of the meat prepared. Take the juice from this quantity—not the broth, but the beef juice. This will give strength, this will assimilate, this will allay, it will destroy the destructive forces in the body, the circulation, and the lungs.   2978-1

For a female adult with incoordination problems between assimilations and eliminations (reading given on March 1, 1937):

Take a pound to a pound and a half preferably of the round steak. No fat, no portions other than that which is of the muscle or tendon for strength; no fatty or skin portions. Dice this into half inch cubes, as it were, or practically so. Put same in a glass jar without water in same. Put the jar then into a boiler or container with the water coming about half or three fourths toward the top of the jar, you see. Preferably put a cloth in the container to prevent the jar from cracking. Do not seal the jar tight, but cover the top. Let this boil (the water, with the jar in same) for three to four hours. Then strain off the juice, and the refuse may be pressed somewhat. It will be found that the meat or flesh itself will be worthless. Place the juice in a cool place, but do not keep too long; never longer than three days, see? Hence the quantity made up at the time depends upon how much or how often the body will take this. It should be taken two to three times a day, but not more than a table-spoonful at the time—and this sipped very slowly. Of course, this is to be seasoned to suit the taste of the body.

Well, too, that whole wheat or Ry-Krisp crackers be taken with same to make it more palatable.   1343-2

TESTIMONIALS/RESULTS
Report written by Mrs. H.B. Harrell, Jr., on March 27, 1950:

"Have followed Health Hint {*column in* A.R.E. Bulletin, *an early A.R.E. publication*} many times in taking beef juice 1 teaspoonful three times daily. I feel a definite gain in strength after taking it for one week after having had a cold."   1343-2, Report #5

Excerpt from a letter from Mrs. [1523] written on December 17, 1947, to Gladys Davis:

" . . . when I was home last June—if you remember, I didn't feel so hot—when I came back I didn't pull out of it; nothing I seemed to be able to put my finger on, but just felt depressed and lifeless. So one day when I was talking to a Mr. Lewis . . . about his health, suggesting that he better have his blood pressure checked—it dawned on me that— that was what was wrong with me. I promptly made up my beef juice (a favorite of mine anyhow) and in two weeks' time I felt like a new person. I took two series of beef juice. There is just nothing like it, and it's so pleasant to take . . . "   1523-17, Report #6

Excerpt from a letter from Edgar Cayce to Mrs. [325] regarding her health (several people reported a burning sensation in their throats and mouths when ingesting the beef juice):

"I'm afraid they have been tending to give you too much of the beef juice at a time. There shouldn't be more than a teaspoonful at any time, and it would be much better to be half a teaspoonful. It is true that this tends to make the gastric juices work more regularly in your system, but that's what you need to get rid of those conditions that produce the nausea as well as the irritations caused by the gas and acid.

"It may be the same reason why the concentrated vegetable juices burn; that they have given you too much at once. It's better that you be given a spoonful every half hour to an hour, rather than taking a big swallow two or three times a day."   325-50, Report #2

ADDITIONAL INFORMATION

That beef juice is to be taken as a tonic or as medicine offers a clue as to when one would use it. A number of the readings' recipients were debilitated with a longstanding illness or disease process or they were suffering the aftereffects of surgery; consequently, they were on a liquid or semi-liquid diet, trying to regain their strength and stamina by ingesting easily assimilated and easily digested foods.

The strengthening quality of this food item is frequently noted; for example, " . . . there is more strength and body-building in one spoonful of beef juice than a pound of the raw meat or rare meat or cooked! and the system will build more from same if taken in that way and manner . . . " (1259-2)

A person who needed more calcium in his system was told that " . . . the beef juice—if not in excess—will assist in the general condition for the body, as well as all properties carrying more of those that build muscle, tissue, bone and structural forces of the body." (142-4) It may also be taken when one is feeling tired or weak.

Two recommendations remain consistent throughout the readings in the taking of beef juice: *small amounts* are to be taken each time, and this quantity is always to be *sipped slowly*, taking one's time to swallow it. One reading states: " . . . almost *chew* it—though there is nothing to chew, of course—for it is liquid . . . " (975-5) Two other excerpts follow:

 . . . Give a teaspoonful at the time, but let the body be at least two minutes in sipping that quantity. Let it rather be absorbed than swallowed. Let it just flow with the salivary glands and be absorbed through the body-force by the gentle swallowing. There will be little or none to digest, but will be absorbed.   3316-1

. . . But take at least a teaspoonful of beef juice four times each day
and take at least a minute and a half in sipping this. That is, just sip it
sufficiently that there is scarcely the need for even swallowing but let
it be absorbed in the mouth as well as just trickle, as it were, to the
throat and stomach, and then a swallow . . .   5334-1

Why the Cayce readings' emphasis on sipping the juice? The reason
for this may lie in its high concentration, as noted in several readings.
"If the beef juice is prepared properly, a tablespoonful of this carries *all*
of the elements that are most worth while for the system—as much as
from as large a steak as an ordinary person might eat." (556-8) " . . . A
tablespoon is almost equal to a pound of meat or two pounds of meat
a day; and that's right smart for a man that isn't active!" (1424-2)

The equivalent of a smaller amount of beef juice is expressed in the
following: " . . . A teaspoonful of this is worth much more than a quarter
pound steak. This is worth much more than five pounds of potatoes. It
is worth much more than a whole head of cabbage, unless the cabbage
is eaten raw—and this wouldn't be very well for this body . . . " (667-8)
Sipping it slowly also helps the body to better assimilate it.

In the *Physician's Reference Notebook*, Dr. William McGarey states that
regular use of beef juice has these benefits: "It apparently could bring
about a strengthening of the body without irritating the cells in the
intestinal tract which might bring about a change in the nature of the
lymph and the lymphatic functioning . . . " (p. 374) This idea seems to be
borne out in the information contained in the following reading:

. . . This, sipped in this manner, will work towards producing the gastric flow through the intestinal system, first in the salivary reactions to
the very nature of the properties themselves, second with the gastric
flow from the upper portion of the stomach or through the cardiac reaction at the end of the esophagus that produces the first of the
lacteals' {*lymphatic vessels in the small intestine*} reaction to the gastric flows in the stomach or digestive forces themselves; thirdly mak-

ing for an activity through the pylorus and the duodenum that becomes
stimulating to the activity of the flows without producing the tendencies for accumulation of gases.   1100-10

For those times when one may need some extra energy or vitality, a
small amount of beef juice may be just the right help to get back on
track.

Castor Oil Pack

Many of us may recall a family member—usually elderly— who strongly urged us to swallow some castor oil to maintain regularity; that is, as a preventative for constipation. In addition, there is the wholehearted and enthusiastic endorsement of Dr. William McGarey, who has written and spoken extensively on castor oil's other therapeutic benefits, introducing numerous patients as well as the public to its positive effects. While it is still used today medically as a cathartic, the Cayce readings also recommend external applications for massage and most frequently as a pack, in over five hundred cases.

Castor oil packs are a well-known item in the Cayce pharmacopeia, with at least thirty physiological effects described in the readings and recommended for over fifty ailments. Due to its variety of applications and successful healing results, the frequent advice from A.R.E. headquarters is: "When in doubt, use castor oil!"

INDICATIONS

(For packs) Acidity, adhesions, aphonia, appendicitis, arthritis, cancer, cerebral palsy, cholecystitis, cirrhosis of the liver, colitis, constipation, cysts, diarrhea, epilepsy, fatigue, flatulence, gallstones, gastritis, halitosis (bad breath), headaches, hepatitis, hernias, Hodgkin's disease, hookworm, hypertension, incoordination of the nervous system, inflammation, intestinal impaction, lesions, lymphitis, multiple sclerosis, nausea, neuritis, Parkinson's disease, pelvic cellulitis, poor circulation (blood and lymph), poor eliminations, prolapsis, ringworm, scleroderma, sluggish liver, stenosis of the duodenum, sterility, strangulation of kidneys, stricture of the duodenum, swelling, toxemia, tumors, uremia, vaginal fistulas

(For massages, applied locally) Abrasions, moles, warts, wens; (full body) Epilepsy, ichthyosis (congenital disease producing dry, scaly skin—like a fish)

CONTRAINDICATIONS

Avoid heat (from electric heating pad) if there is unidentified, undiagnosed pain in the abdomen, as heat might exacerbate it or intensify inflammation; do not use heat on the abdomen during pregnancy or with excessive stomach or intestinal gas; several readings state to avoid packs during the menstrual flow

MATERIALS NEEDED

Bottle of pure, cold-pressed castor oil

Wool flannel cloth—large enough piece to cover abdomen after being folded 2 to 4 times

Electric heating pad or hot water bottle

Large piece of plastic, such as a white garbage bag—to place between heating pad and wool flannel pack

Large bath towel—to place over entire pack and hold it in place

Oil cloth, thick towel, or plastic liner—to place on bed to protect sheets

Baking soda (1 teaspoon) and warm water (1 pint) plus wash cloth—to wipe oil off abdomen after pack is removed

Olive oil (small amounts)—to take orally after last castor oil pack in series is taken

Plastic container or glass jar—to store pack in cool place when finished using it

FREQUENCY OF APPLICATION

(For packs) Daily; every other day; 1 to 2 days, rest for 1 week, repeat; 2 or 3 days, rest 2 or 3 days—duration for 10 days; 3 days in a row; 2 to 3 days, rest a week, then repeat; 3, 4, or 5 days; 5 to 10 days, leave off 3, 4, or 5 days; 5 days, rest 3 days, repeat; 2 or 3 times a week; 3 days a week for 3 to 4 weeks; 8 to 10 days; once a month; 3 to 4 weeks

(For full-body massages) Once a week; 3 days in succession; (for local application for hands and fingers) Daily

AMOUNT OF DOSAGE OF OLIVE OIL

After 3-day series of castor oil packs take ½ teaspoon 3 to 4 times a day for 2 to 3 days, then following second 3-day series of packs take 1 teaspoon 2 to 3 times daily for 2 days; ¼ to ½ teaspoon 3 to 4 times daily; 1 teaspoon 2 to 4 times daily; 2 teaspoons (or 1 teaspoon twice a day); 1 or 2 tablespoons; " . . . all the body will assimilate, but not in large quantities at the dose—rather the very small quantities taken often." (704-1); " . . . a quantity of Olive Oil—just so it is not sufficient to cause regurgitation or vomiting . . . " (1553-7); half a teacup (1 teacup holds about 3 to 8 fluid ounces)

Note: Only a few readings mention taking the olive oil on the same days as the packs.

Caution: With liver or gall bladder problems, take olive oil sparingly—only the minimum amount.

WHEN TO TAKE THE CASTOR OIL PACK

Before or after osteopathic treatments; before a colonic; " . . . when there are upsettings in the liver area . . . " (3050-2); "When there is acute pain through the abdomen . . . " (3043-1)—if undiagnosed, avoid heat

LENGTH OF TIME OF APPLICATION

One-half hour to 1 hour; 1 hour to 1½ hours; 2, 3, 4, 5, 6, or 7 hours; " . . . kept up for a period sufficient to produce a reaction . . . " (5449-3); "Until the eliminations are correctly established . . . " (348-19); continuously until pain ceases; all evening or all night

LOCATION OF APPLICATION

(For packs) Across abdomen, right and left sides; across the area of the lacteal ducts, spleen, pancreas, liver, caecum; appendicial area; area below the diaphragm; cardiac portion of stomach and lower abdomen; extending around the body, left side; gall duct; jejunum; lower portion of right rib; stomach and duodenum; toward the back; umbilicus plexus (right side)

(For scleroderma) Neck, shoulders, hips, lower limbs—" . . . any portion where this hardening occurs . . . " (528-8); " . . . where the skin is affected . . . " (2514-3); calf of leg, around the arms, and across the back of the shoulders

(For massages with the oil, applied locally) Cheek or lip abrasions, mole on chest, protruding bone near elbow, stiff hands and fingers, warts, wen (benign skin tumor) above the eye; (full-body massages) Abdomen, back, diaphragm area, feet; " . . . along the whole length of the cerebrospinal system . . . " (1385-1)

SIZE OF PACK

Large enough to fit over specific abdominal area after wool flannel has been folded 2 to 4 thicknesses; 16 to 18 inches square (41 cm to 46 cm) (4299-2)

EXPECTED EFFECTS/PURPOSES

Increases eliminations and lymphatic circulation

Stimulates the liver, gall bladder, lacteal duct circulation, and peristalsis

Dissolves and removes lesions, adhesions (in the lacteal duct), and tumors

Relieves pain and headaches and increases relaxation

Reduces toxemia, inflammation, flatulence, nausea, nervous system incoordination, and swelling

Dissolves gallstones and balances eliminations

Improves gastrointestinal assimilation, perspiration–respiration coordination, and liver–kidney coordination

Releases colon impaction

Stimulates the cecum, organs, and glands

Draws out acids and discharge from vaginal fistulas

Increases skin circulation (blood and lymph)

DIRECTIONS

The material recommended for the pack is wool flannel, folded two to four thicknesses and large enough to adequately cover the area of application. The oil is to be heated beforehand. Why? One reading explained: " . . . this heating breaks the atomic forces in the oil so that it is more penetrating to the body when applied to same . . . " (4299-2) In a note attached to reading 623-3, Gladys Davis, Cayce's secretary, wrote: " . . . Dip the flannel in hot Castor Oil and apply as hot as may be stood; keep them hot during the whole three-hour period each treatment. This is so the pores of the skin are opened and as much oil as possible is allowed to soak in."

One way to heat this oil is to first place the wool flannel on a piece of plastic wrap, pour castor oil on the cloth (so that it is well saturated but not dripping), and then set both pieces on an electric heating pad turned on low. The plastic wrap protects the pad. After it has warmed up, lie down on a plastic sheet, towel, or covering to protect your bed sheets. Place the wool flannel directly on your skin over the abdomen, usually on the liver/gall duct area (right side), followed by the plastic coating, the heating pad, and finally a large bath towel, folded lengthwise, covering all the layers and tucked in around the sides of your body.

Switch the pad to a medium or high setting. Now spend the next hour or so in quiet prayer, meditation, or inspirational reading. It's easy to doze off, so you might want to set an alarm to awaken at the appropriate time. Then remove the pack, sponge off the area with a baking soda and water solution, and, if this pack is the last of the series, take your dose of olive oil. (Only a few readings recommend taking the olive oil on the same days as the packs.)

Each time the pack is removed, the area is sponged off with a weak solution of baking soda and warm water ("soda water") " . . . to remove the oil or the excess accumulations produced by the heat . . . " (2920-1) Several readings mention the acidity of castor oil, so the baking soda

" . . . is needed to produce a reaction of an alkaline nature in the body."
(3367-1) Amounts in the recipe varied slightly. A weak solution, for example, would be about a teaspoon of baking soda to a pint of warm
water.

After one finishes applying the final castor oil pack in the series, olive
oil is to be consumed; recommendations on amounts range from one-
fourth teaspoon to half a teacup (one teacup equals about three to eight
fluid ounces). This taking of oil helps with assimilation and acts " . . . as
a food as well as an eliminant for the alimentary canal." (1553-7) Digest-
ing it also increases bile flow from both the liver and gall bladder; thus,
according to Dr. Harold Reilly, if one has gall bladder or liver problems,
the olive oil should be taken sparingly, consuming only the minimum
amount.

When not in use, store the pack in a glass jar or heavy plastic container and keep it in a cool place. The oil is fairly stable, not turning
rancid quickly, allowing the pack to be reused even up to several years.
Add a small fresh layer (about one tablespoon) of castor oil, though,
onto the pack before each reuse. Of course, if the oil has turned rancid
or the pack has become soiled, discard.

DIRECTIONS FROM THE READINGS

For a fifteen-year-old girl suffering from poor eliminations, cholecystitis (inflammation or infection of the gall bladder), and abrasions
(reading given on June 8, 1932):

> First we would begin with this: Each evening, over the liver area, apply
> Castor Oil packs. Take a square of flannel that is three-ply, at least, in
> its thickness, that is at least sixteen to eighteen inches square. This
> we would thoroughly saturate by dipping in Castor Oil, and have the oil
> as hot as can be borne on the body. This should be put next to the skin.
> Do not attempt to put on cold and then heat with pack, or with electric
> pads, but rather have the oil as hot as may be from the *heating* of the
> oil itself; for this heating breaks the atomic forces in the oil so that it is
> more penetrating to the body when applied to same. This may be left
> on for the whole evening or night, see? One heating will be sufficient,

if there will be used heavy packs that will prevent this becoming too messy, or too much losing of the effect of that obtained in the pack by the dipping and wringing out of same. This pack should cover the liver area, especially—more to the umbilicii center and then backward, see, over the right side. This should cover the area especially of the lacteal ducts, the pancrean area and the gall duct area, which lies between the two lobes—and especially toward the center, a span from the umbilicii center, up and to the right, see?

In the morning sponge off this area of the body with soda water, which will cleanse and also open the pores.

The next evening we would do the same. This we would keep up for at least eight to ten days, see?

On the fifth day, begin with small doses of olive oil taken internally, all the body will assimilate—but take in very small doses, three or four times each day a quarter to half a teaspoonful of pure olive oil. Should this become rancid, then reduce the quantity but continue to take same.   4299-2

[Note that in this reading the olive oil is taken before the eight-to-ten-day series of packs is completed.]

For a sixty-year-old woman with arthritis and cholecystitis (reading given on September 5, 1943):

We would begin applying Castor Oil Packs for an hour each day, for three days in succession; not so hot as to cause too great a discomfort, but so that the area will receive—as it were—a baptism of oil as will be absorbed in the activity of the area about the liver and gall duct. Use at least three thicknesses of flannel thoroughly saturated with the Castor Oil, applied over the liver and gall duct area. Use oil cloth over same to protect the linens, and then an electric pad to keep same warm for at least an hour, at low heat.

When removing the Pack, sponge off the area with a weak soda water solution.

On the evening of the third day, following the taking of the third

Castor Oil Pack, take internally two tablespoonsful of Olive Oil.
Then rest from these applications for five days.   3196-1

TESTIMONIALS/RESULTS

A letter dated June 29, 1975, written by an A.R.E. member from Yon-
kers, New York, Mrs. Richard T. Brand, contained this information:

"I have just finished reading an article from the July *A.R.E. Journal*
{*former membership publication which later became* Venture Inward
magazine} entitled 'Laying On of Hands.' The story was very signifi-
cant for me because I had an experience similar to that woman. I too
had discovered a lump in my breast and was told to see a surgeon as
soon as possible. My doctor told me he thought it was a cyst and not a
tumor, but in any event should be removed.

"I had read where Castor Oil Packs on external cysts, warts, and
moles were beneficial but I hadn't read where it was recommended for
the breast. Well, I applied the packs faithfully for about a week. I even
fell asleep once with a pack on! Almost immediately the size of the
lump decreased. During this time I meditated daily. I say this only because I often miss a day or two and I know meditation has a healing
effect on the body.

"During the next month I continued the packs but only once every
two days.

"It is now two months later since finding the lump and it has disappeared. I returned to my doctor and after examining me found every-
thing normal. He asked if I saw the surgeon and I replied, 'No.'
Whatever—the lump is gone and I feel the Castor Oil had a lot to do
with it."   683-3, Report #4

A surgeon in Shillington, Pennsylvania, Dr. Bob McTammany, related
the following story to Dr. William McGarey, who writes in *The Oil That
Heals*:

"He told me . . . about a post-vaginal hysterectomy patient who developed a febrile course and a large pelvic abscess which improved on

antibiotics and proteolytic enzymes, although a 10 x 10 cm mass remained. She refused further surgery, and after several weeks of malaise, fever, low abdominal tenderness and pain, and no general improvement, she was then convinced that she should begin application of castor oil packs, used one hour daily. She improved remarkably symptom-wise, and examination in one month showed almost complete resolution of the pelvic abscess. Bob feels that these packs might be beneficial to post-operative patients in order to improve wound healing and reduce the incidence of infection."

From a research report by a woman correspondent who wrote to the A.R.E. Clinic in Phoenix, Arizona (no longer in operation), comes this story, later submitted by Dr. William McGarey to "Notes from the Medical Research Bulletin" in *The A.R.E. Journal*:

"An alcoholic for more than 20 years . . . she used castor oil packs on her abdomen for an entirely different reason four years ago. It seemed that she had developed a severe abdominal pain. She did not consult her doctor, so her own diagnosis of 'probably an intestinal disorder' will have to suffice, no matter how inadequate. She reports that her pain lessened a little each day, as she applied the packs on a twice daily routine. An apparent constipation was thoroughly corrected on the second day, but she continued the packs for a period of two weeks.

"The most remarkable result of her own little adventure in consciousness, however, is the real point of this story. She adds as a postscript to her report that 'Since the day I first used oil packs, I have not touched a drop of liquor—nor have I had the desire to do so . . . I used to drink myself to sleep every single night.'

"My question is: What is it that happens to people that makes a simple act of healing turn their lives into a new channel of living? Why should applications of castor oil packs rival Alcoholics Anonymous in this particular event in time and space? Life offers us a multitude of unanswered questions, doesn't it?"

Further accounts of individuals' experiences with castor oil can be found in Dr. William A. McGarey's book *The Oil That Heals* and David E. Kukor's book *The Miracle Oil* (both published by A.R.E. Press).

ADDITIONAL INFORMATION

What exactly is castor oil? It is a yellowish–colored oil that is extracted from the castor bean or seed of the *Ricinus communis,* a tall tropical plant with large palmate leaves, also known as *Palma Christi* (palm of Christ). The castor oil plant is native to India, where it has been used extensively to treat all types of gastrointestinal disorders, bladder and vaginal infections, and asthma. In Russia it is used as a lubricant in industrial equipment because of its consistent viscosity; it won't freeze even in Russia's severe winters. It is also used there medicinally to restore hair and to treat constipation, eye irritations, and skin ulcers.

Chemically, castor oil is a triglyceride of fatty acids, nearly ninety percent of which is an unsaturated fatty acid called ricinoleic acid. (Triglycerides play an important role in metabolism as energy sources.) It is thought that the high concentration of this ingredient gives the oil its remarkable healing qualities. Ricinoleic acid has been shown to be effective in preventing the growth of various species of bacteria, yeast, molds, and viruses (Novak, A.F., et al., *Journal of the American Oil Chemists' Society,* 1961, No. 37, pp. 323–325). Perhaps this quality accounts for its high success rate in topical applications and antimicrobial activity.

Cayce offers another perspective in the following two extracts:

> ... Consider that which takes place from the use of the oil pack and its influence upon the body, and something of the emotion experienced may be partially understood.
>
> Oil is that which constitutes, in a form, the nature of activity between the functionings of the organs of the system; as related to activity. Much in the same manner as upon an inanimate object it acts as a limbering agent, or allowing movement, motion, as may be had by the attempt to move a hinge, a wrench, a center, or that movement of an inanimate machinery motion. This is the same effect had upon that which is now animated by spirit. This movement, then, was the reflection of the abilities of the spiritual of *animate* activity as controlled

through the emotions of mind, or the activity of mind between spirit
and matter . . .   1523-15

(Q) Should the Castor Oil packs still be taken?
(A) When necessary for the proper eliminations to be carried on in
system; nothing will be found better, for this aids the organs in their
necessary overactivity in eliminating the character of drosses created
by the destruction of bacilli that will be carried on, and that is being
carried on in the system. Do not allow the bowels or the colon to become clogged. Keep the eliminations properly. This is better done by
either the diet or by outside influences than by poisoning or overtax-
ing the muco-membranes of the digestive system, by creating excite-
ment to the activity of the lymph and emunctory circulation, or by
taking cathartics or purgatives.   325-43

OTHER USES FOR CASTOR OIL

The introductory paragraph to this chapter mentions that there are
other uses for castor oil. In addition to packs, the readings suggest its
use in enemas, for massages, and the traditional remedy of taking it
orally as a laxative. Here is one example of castor oil in an **enema:**

. . . we would first begin with small enemas of as hot Castor Oil as the
body can stand. Not that this is to be so warm or hot as to cause such a
great discomfort but sufficiently warm that it may be injected with a
pumping enema—about two or three tablespoonful{*s*}. Give these
about every other day.   1375-1

For **massages** there are only a few references to using castor oil as a
lubricant, mentioning that it might be a bit messy. Castor oil does stain
sheets and clothing, so precautions may need to be taken to avoid stain-
ing. Some readings mention specific areas to be massaged; for example,
" . . . along the whole length of the cerebrospinal system . . . " (1385–1)
Other readings suggest only local applications, such as on warts, abrasions, moles, and wens.

In the following two excerpts as an eliminant or a **laxative**, each one mentions another substance to be taken with the oil:

> (Q) Should I take the Castor Oil?
> (A) As an eliminant, very good eliminant! Necessary after taking such
> an eliminant that there be either Syrup of Figs or Castoria taken to
> *tone* the system without making a strain from the overacidity produced
> in the alimentary canal.   288-39

> Castor oil should be taken as an *eliminant,* followed by any saline that
> cleanses same from system—and should be at least three to five days
> apart in doses taken, see? taking about tablespoonful to tablespoonful
> and a half at a dose, followed with that of a mild saline the next morn-
> ing.
>   The *olive* oil should be a teaspoonful once each day.
>   Now the effect of these on the system: We find the castor oil in its
> reaction is an acid. Hence that of the saline following same to cleanse
> the system, yet the system needs that of the excitement to the mucus
> coating of the duodenum, the activity of liver, and the reduction of the
> forces in the spleen's reaction with digestive forces, as well as the
> cleansing of the lower intestinal tract. The olive oil is a food for the
> intestinal system when taken in small doses. *Do* that.   195-58

From a country doctor quoted by Dr. William McGarey comes this
excellent summary statement of the oil's beneficial healing effects: "Castor oil will leave the body in better condition than it found it."

Charred Oak Keg

The charred oak keg is a rather unusual, unique remedy recommended to over eighty individuals who presented their health concerns to Cayce. From one reading to another the size of the keg varies only slightly: a container able to hold from one to five gallons, filled with a smaller proportion of pure apple brandy, described as " . . . brandy that has been redistilled . . . " (4018-1) or " . . . double distilled apple brandy . . . " (3222-1) or " . . . pure distilled apple brandy . . . " (5239-1)—not applejack. Laird's is the brand recommended today. Fumes that arise from this brandy are then inhaled through a tube or opening on the top of the keg for a variety of respiratory conditions.

The wooden keg consists of oak, with its interior charred or burnt. The charcoal from this inside surface absorbs impurities from the liquor stored within it; hence, these kegs are used commercially to store aging liquors. " . . . The char in the charred surfaces of the oak barrels is actually a form of activated charcoal which . . . {is} an absorber of impurities." (5374-1, Report #10) This absorptive property may be the reason Cayce recommends keeping the brandy in this type of keg.

Instructions in the readings describe installing two vents or tubes—

a smaller one to assist the air pressure and help prevent a vacuum, and a large hole inserted with a tube of rubber, glass, or metal in order to inhale the fumes from the brandy. Both vents remain corked when the keg is not in use. The inhalation tube rests slightly above the liquid brandy. Kegs purchased today, however, conveniently have for inhalation just one vent or hole that is kept plugged with a cork when not in use.

Directions for the keg were usually included with each individual's reading. Since the charred oak keg is now available from the official worldwide supplier of Cayce products, it can be purchased and is ready for immediate use after a few instructions are followed and the brandy is added.

INDICATIONS

Asthma, colds, coughs, hay fever, lung congestion, other respiratory ailments (bronchiectasis, bronchitis, chronic obstructive pulmonary disease, emphysema, fibrosis, nasal drip, pneumonia, sarcoidosis, smoker's lung), pleurisy, shortness of breath, tuberculosis or TB tendencies

CONTRAINDICATIONS

Do not inhale brandy fumes from the charred oak keg on the same day you are using the Violet Ray device

MATERIALS NEEDED

Wooden keg of oak, with its interior charred or burnt

Tube of rubber, glass, or metal to inhale fumes from brandy—supplied with keg

Pure 100–proof apple brandy (Laird's is the recommended brand today)

Round cork to seal the openings or opening when not in use—supplied with keg

Colander or screen—to place over opening when preparing or cleansing the keg

FREQUENCY OF APPLICATION
Once or twice a day inhale the fumes, then after a few weeks 3 times a day, inhaling 2 or 3 times at each period; 2, 3, or 4 times daily; " . . . The frequency of the inhaling will be governed by the reaction . . . " (929-1)

AMOUNT OF APPLICATION
A few small whiffs in the beginning 1 or 2 times daily, then 3, 4, or 5 inhalations at each session, " . . . as one would inhale smoke from a cigarette . . . " (2395-1)

LENGTH OF TIME OF APPLICATION
Daily; 3 to 10 minutes; use 3 to 4 days, off 1 week to 10 days, then repeat; at least 2 weeks; use when feeling shaky, weak, or " . . . when there is a great deal of wet or cold weather and the tendency for cold or congestion is prevalent." (421-13)

SIZE OF KEG
Varied sizes (in gallons): 1, 1½, 2, 2½, 3, or 5; *ratio of size of keg to amount of brandy*: 1-gallon keg: ½ gallon of brandy; 1½-gallon keg: ½ or ¾ gallon of brandy; 1½- or 2-gallon keg: 1 gallon of brandy; 2-gallon keg: 3 quarts of brandy; 2- or 3-gallon keg: 1 or 1½ gallons of brandy

EXPECTED EFFECTS/PURPOSES
Destroys live tubercle tissue
Acts as an antiseptic for irritated areas
Stimulates circulation
Increases the abilities of assimilation
Allays coughing and other irritations
Purifies lung tissue
Eliminates infection
Prevents inflamed mucous membranes
Lessens the effect of acidity on the body
Prevents " . . . the body from so easily taking cold . . . " (357-9)

DIRECTIONS

Preparing the keg involves tightening the metal bands as much as possible beforehand, then unplugging the vent hole and placing the entire keg in warm water, filling the inside completely with distilled water and allowing it to soak for two to three days. This soaking causes the wooden keg to swell and expand, sealing the seams and preventing leakage later when the brandy is poured in.

After the soaking period, place a screen over the hole and pour out the water through the screen, thus keeping any loose charcoal chips in the keg. The brandy can now be added, an amount roughly one-half the size of the keg. Let it sit overnight, and the next day it is ready for use.

Warm the keg slightly [about 85° F (29.4° C)]—by placing it in warm water or next to a radiator; near a heating vent, stove, or heater; in the sunlight; or simply wrap a large heating pad around the keg. This warmth induces evaporation. One reading clarifies the amount of heat: " . . . not so much as to cause the Brandy to evaporate too fast, but {keep it} in a warm place . . . " (2183-2) Next, open the vent by removing the cork. Now the fumes from the brandy can be inhaled through the mouth and/or the nose.

The readings caution against inhaling too much at the beginning, as " . . . it will be inclined to produce too much intoxication for the body." (2448-1) Gradually increase the inhalations, taking in 1 or 2 whiffs at first, then later in up to 3, 4, or 5 sessions a day, taking 1 to 5 whiffs each time.

At a health fair displaying Cayce-related items, the guidance for each person who used the keg was to first take a deep breath and then exhale fully. Remove the cork, place your mouth on the tube or over the vent opening (the sides of the hole were wrapped with a protective covering and replaced for each person), and inhale deeply. The fumes from the brandy go directly into the lungs through the mouth, larynx, and throat. Some individuals were told in their readings to inhale through the nasal passages as well.

The keg may be kept warm " . . . so that evaporation may occur easily." (3154-1) Then it is ready for your next inhalation or for a follow-up session later. You may choose to remove the heating pad or turn it off until just prior to your next session. Whenever there is not enough of a fume for the next inhalation, shake the keg a little to stir up the brandy. The fumes from the brandy heal lung tissue by destroying live tubercle cells, stimulating circulation, allaying coughing and other irritations, and preventing the mucous membranes from becoming inflamed.

Caring for the keg involves cleansing it and replacing the brandy, as well as adding to the brandy when its level is low. One reading stated: " . . . Do not let the brandy get too low. When it has evaporated to half or two-thirds of the quantity, refill . . . " (3176-1) When there are almost no fumes at all arising from the keg, it is time to recharge it by rinsing it out and replacing the liquor. Using a colander, pour the contents of the keg down the sink, retaining the bits of charcoal. Rinse the keg well with warm water, again pouring the liquid through the colander. Then replace the charcoal bits into the keg and add fresh brandy. One reading explains the reason for this procedure:

> . . . Rinse with *warm*—not hot but *warm* water, so that the accumulations from the distillation or evaporation of the properties are removed, and there is less of that influence or force which arises from the acids that come from such infusions.   1548-4

In a letter to Mr. [3085] dated January 15, 1944, Cayce wrote: " . . . you will have to discard that that has been in the keg until you have been using it for nearly twelve months . . . " (3085-2, Report #3)

DIRECTIONS FROM THE READINGS

For a twenty-four-year-old female bookkeeper suffering from respiratory weakness, poor lungs, and a susceptibility to colds (reading given on February 8, 1941):

> As an inhalant we would use the fume from Apple Brandy. Do not drink the brandy, but inhale the fumes from same. Prepare this in a keg—a charred oak keg—so that the fumes may be inhaled; having two holes

in one end, but so that they may be kept tightly corked except when being used—and open when there is the inhaling of the fumes from the Brandy. Put half a gallon of Apple Brandy—*not* Applejack—in about a gallon container. Keep where it will be easy for the evaporation to take place, or for the gases to form in the space above the Brandy, you see. When the fumes are inhaled, it will act not only as a purifier for the throat, bronchi and lungs, but will be a stimulation to the circulation. Use this at least once or twice each day. Do not attempt to inhale too much in the beginning, or it will be inclined to produce too much intoxication for the body.   2448-1

For an adult female with scarred lungs, some hemorrhaging, and tuberculosis tendencies (reading given on March 2, 1922):

Take a three gallon keg, oak that is charred or what is known as whiskey keg, we would put one gallon of apple brandy in this. This is sealed or corked, then set on end and placed close to a heat, where this heat will cause gas to collect in upper portion of the keg. Connect a tube to this and inhale the gas in the larynx and lungs, three or four times a day. Inhale it as would smoke, you see, into mouth, through larynx and in lungs. The first time this is done do not take too much or it will produce intoxication to the sensories. It will carry the healing properties.   3354-1

For a twenty–eight–year–old woman suffering with moderately advanced tuberculosis for six and one–half years (reading given on March 27, 1944):

Also begin inhaling the fumes from pure apple brandy in a charred oak keg, prepared with two vents in one end. This should be redistilled brandy. Do not swallow the fumes into the stomach but inhale into the lungs. Do not let the inhalations be too heavy in the beginning, else we may cause some disturbance to the coughing and the raw area in the left lung, as well as sore areas in the trachea on the right side. But as these fumes are inhaled, they will cause the destruction of active tissue and, if the other properties are added, the sputum will soon become negative and less active.   4024-1

TESTIMONIALS/RESULTS

In the "Reports" section of the readings not many testimonials are found. Most of the correspondence deals with questions on where to obtain the keg or the apple brandy. Yet scattered throughout are comments on the efficacy of the keg, especially for tuberculosis, that were reported back to Cayce and his small staff. One such comment comes from a letter dated August 17, 1943, from Mrs. [2395], who received only one reading three years earlier:

> "It looks like I am always sending out an S.O.S. to you. Do you suppose you could get me any pure Apple Brandy out there and send it to me! I can't get any here {in Kentucky}, and with Hay Fever just around the corner I would like very much to be prepared to fight it . . . As you may probably remember, in your reading of November 8, 1940, you prescribed the Apple Brandy to be inhaled from a charred oak keg and I feel that it was very beneficial . . . "   2395-1, Report #7

Cayce wrote a few days later that due to war conditions it was impossible to obtain the brandy.

Perhaps the most well-known account of the keg's use comes from the Cayce family itself. Gertrude, Edgar's wife, distraught after the death of her almost two-month-old son, Milton Porter, stopped eating and spent much of her time in bed. Two months later she was coughing up blood. The diagnosis: tuberculosis, a disease that had previously claimed the life of her brother. Her eventual reading in 1911 contained, among other suggestions, the remedy of inhaling brandy fumes from a charred oak keg. Gertrude followed the suggestions, and her lungs eventually became less congestive. It was a slow process, but finally Gertrude was healed.

ADDITIONAL INFORMATION

In March 2000, the Heritage Store in Virginia Beach, VA, sent out a brief questionnaire to people who had purchased a charred oak keg within the last few years. Twenty-nine individuals responded. While the majority of recommendations from the Cayce readings concerned those with tuberculosis or TB tendencies—with a few cases of asthma, pleurisy, and various lung problems—a wider range of respiratory ailments was noted by the survey responders: bronchiectasis, bronchitis, chronic cough, chronic obstructive pulmonary disease, colds, congestion, emphysema, fibrosis, nasal drip, pneumonia, sarcoidosis, and smoker's lung. Several even used it to help quit smoking and others to achieve better athletic performance.

In rating their success with the keg, consistency of use seemed to be the main factor influencing a better outcome; those individuals using it on a regular basis reported good or better results.

Some of the differences noted by the survey participants included: coughing less often, breathing more easily, and experiencing a decrease in the number of colds and respiratory infections, the loosening up of congestion, as well as the alleviation of pain. One individual, taking oxygen for emphysema and chronic bronchitis, commented that inhaling from the keg "loosens mucus to cough up, expel; medicates lung and bronchi, keeping down infections."

Remedial use of the keg was found to be effective at the onset of congestion to help cough up mucus, when losing one's voice, and to open breathing passages. Another individual, susceptible to colds, noted: "I took so many antibiotics that I became allergic to two of them, so the charred oak keg was always a rescue mission for me." Two respondents commented that the keg helped reduce their desire to smoke; one mentioned taking a whiff from the keg each time the urge to light up arose. Another used it "to enhance oxygen intake for extreme sports training."

With proper care and use, the keg can be a healing influence on the lungs. One excerpt succinctly stated: "Keep the *keg*. This *is* as life itself . . . " (1548-4)

Coffee Foot Bath

Foot baths are one of the most useful and easily applied hydrotherapies. Requiring only a minimal amount of equipment, the foot bath can be accomplished while seated on a chair, a sofa, or on the edge of the bathtub. A foot tub may be purchased, but one may use any basin or pan that is waterproof and encloses the feet comfortably.

Eleven individuals were given this very specific kind of foot bath: it is made with used coffee grounds that are boiled just prior to the bath, letting the solution cool a bit before soaking the feet in the warm mixture. This mild tannic acid solution, derived from coffee, has beneficial effects, according to the readings, when applied *externally*.

Tannin or tannic acid is a yellowish astringent solution whose designation is generic for a wide assortment of vegetable products that are used to tan raw hides, converting them into leather—hence its name. Tannic acid is responsible for coffee's sharp, bitter taste, as well as for causing stained teeth and cups. When drunk, it has been recognized for its harmful effects such as inhibiting the body's absorption of calcium and B vitamins, causing heartburn, acid reflux,

61

and indigestion, interacting with a wide range of medications—reducing their effectiveness—and in large doses causing cancer in animals. Yet its application externally, as mentioned previously, has important and useful benefits.

INDICATIONS

Cold and congestion; heaviness in throat, head, and feet; need for better rest; peeling skin on feet; poor circulation; poor eliminations; tiredness; weak foot arches; OK to apply during menstrual flow

CONTRAINDICATIONS

Check heat tolerance; diabetics or people with poor circulation in feet need to be cautious of water temperature

MATERIALS NEEDED

Small tub, wide bucket, or large pan—to place feet in

Used coffee grounds (not over a day old)—amounts range from 1 to 6 teacups

Pot to boil the used coffee grounds; *ratio of amount of grounds to amount of water*: 1 teacup of grounds: ½ gallon water; 1 cup: 1 or 1½ gallons; 2 cups: 1 to 1½ gallons; 2 to 3 cups: 1 to 1½ gallons; 6 cups: " . . . sufficient water for a good foot bath . . . " (2268-1); " . . . sufficient {grounds} that the water is colored well from the hardboiled coffee grounds." (243-33)

Towels (optional)—to place around tub to protect floor from drips

Bath towel (optional)—to dry off feet after soaking

FREQUENCY OF APPLICATION

Occasionally; daily; each evening before retiring; 1, 2, 3, or 4 times a week; until the cold dissipates

LENGTH OF TIME TO BOIL GROUNDS

Two to 2½ minutes, 10 minutes, 20 to 30 minutes, some readings mention no time length

LENGTH OF TIME OF APPLICATION
Five to 10 minutes, 20 minutes, no time frame given in most readings

LOCATION OF APPLICATION
Lower limbs—feet and ankles; heels, arches, toes, and bottoms of the feet; you can bathe and massage limbs up to the knees with the solution while feet are soaking

EXPECTED EFFECTS/PURPOSES
Enhances circulation
Relieves cold and congestion
Improves functioning of feet

DIRECTIONS
Collect the used coffee grounds from your coffee pot or filter. The grounds should be rather fresh—not over a day old. The amount of coffee grounds ranges from 1 teacup up to 6 cups. Boil the grounds in water from 2 minutes up to 20 to 30 minutes. The amount of water to be boiled ranges from ½ gallon to 1½ gallons. (For the recommended ratio of grounds to amount of water see *Materials Needed* section.)

After the water has been boiling for the specified length of time, allow it to cool somewhat, until it reaches a warm enough temperature (not hot or tepid), so that the feet and lower limbs can be comfortably placed in the water. The grounds may be kept in the water, and the whole solution poured into the foot tub. (Some readings say to strain or remove the grounds; others say not to.) Bathe and massage the feet and lower limbs, using both the water and the grounds (if not strained) as a lubricant, from five to twenty minutes. To do a thorough job, the limbs and knees may be continuously massaged—as well as the heels, arches, toes, and bottoms of the feet—while the feet are soaking. Then dry off the feet and limbs with a towel.

DIRECTIONS FROM THE READINGS
For a twenty-year-old woman who questioned what could be done for the weak arches in her feet (reading given on October 25, 1933):

> . . . Each evening before retiring, bathe the feet and limbs to the knees in a very mild tannic acid, which may best be made (for such conditions) from coffee grounds. When they are ready to be thrown out, put on a cupful to a gallon and a half of water. Let boil for ten minutes, pour off and allow to cool sufficiently so that the lower limbs may be bathed in it. Massage the limbs and the feet, especially the heels and the arches and toes, all the time they are in the solution, see? The whole quantity being used, of course; drain the dregs off, or the grounds; and keep the limbs and feet in same for twenty minutes . . .   386-3

For a thirteen-year-old girl experiencing peeling of the skin on her heels, ankles, and soles of feet (reading given on November 12, 1941):

> . . . Bathe them {*the feet*} occasionally in weak coffee made from old coffee grounds; coffee that has been used, see? Save the old coffee grounds, not until they are soured, but boil and then bathe the feet and lower limbs in same; massaging them with same. Use about a teacup of coffee grounds to half a gallon of water, see? It is the tannic forces from these that has the beneficial effect . . .   2084-10

TESTIMONIALS/RESULTS

A twenty-three-year-old woman who received a total of fifteen readings had anemia, tuberculosis tendencies, and was susceptible to colds. A number of family members also received readings. On October 24, 1933, five days after getting her eighth reading, [421]'s aunt [340] wrote this report on her niece:

> " . . . The reading is excellent, and she needed it very badly. Her mother rubbed her feet and legs as you suggested, last night, and sister [243] said that [421] slept more peacefully than any night for the last three weeks . . . Isn't that coffee grounds suggestion a new one? I'm sure I never heard {*of*} it before, but it does the work."   421-8, Report #2

Report from A.R.E. member, Vincent C. Belton, in Seaford, N.Y., on October 9, 1978, which was placed as a supplement to reading 944-1:

" . . . In May I sent for the {*Circulating*} File on cancer and phlebitis. Why phlebitis? One week after receiving the Circulating File my mother, seventy-nine years young, came down with phlebitis. We proceeded to make up the mullein tea and old coffee grounds extract to apply to her leg. {*She also took a Sal Hepatica series as an intestinal cleanser, as well as 2,000 mg. of vitamin C, 25 mg. of B-6, and 100 mg. of pantothenic acid every two hours.*} Six weeks later her phlebitis was gone along with most of her varicose veins that she has had for as long as I can remember."   944-1, Report #1

ADDITIONAL INFORMATION

After taking the coffee grounds foot bath, instead of immediately drying off the feet, several readings suggested an additional treatment. One sixty–year–old woman was told to follow up her foot bath with a peanut oil massage to her knees, lower legs, and feet. She had complained of being unsteady on her feet and asked for suggestions to relieve her sore, tender feet. Her reading stated that " . . . if this is done consistently, we will relieve these tensions." (243-33)

A thirty–four–year–old woman, suffering from dysmenorrhea, was advised after her foot bath to " . . . massage the cerebrospinal system with an equal combination of Mutton Tallow, Spirits of Turpentine and Spirits of Camphor—perhaps a tablespoonful of the Mutton Tallow (melted), and a tablespoonful of each of the other ingredients, mixed thoroughly together . . . " (2268-1) It could be made fresh each time or a quantity could be made for several uses.

Why should one use coffee grounds that have already been used? Cayce clarified what he meant by fresh, yet used grounds:

. . . a solution {*is*} made from used coffee grounds; not soured grounds, but fresh—that is, not over a day old after being first used, see? Not the fresh coffee; it is preferable to use the grounds, that have the more tannin in same. Consequently the *used* grounds are preferable . . . The quantity of tannic acid from this source is preferable to using tannic acid in other solutions to massage. And the massaging with this solution, with the grounds in same, will stimulate the circulation . . .   2315-1

OTHER USES FOR COFFEE GROUNDS

Massaging the scalp with old coffee grounds not only " . . . would keep the hair colored but it would be effective to make same grow." (2301-5) This information was given to a thirty–one–year–old man who was having his fifth reading on August 27, 1943.

An insurance agent, a thirty–seven–year–old male, on October 31, 1942, had a similar request: "How may I promote the growth of new hair on my head? . . . " The reading advised: " . . . Eat more shell fish; and rub same with a few coffee grounds occasionally." (2533-6)

For a sixteen–year–old girl receiving her seventh reading from Cayce on April 14, 1934, who asked, "What is the best formula that will make my skin brown from the sun?" this reply was offered:

> . . . Sun tan for some is good. But for those that have a certain amount of pigment in the skin, as indicated in this body, to make for variations as to the effect of weather or sun upon exposed portions of the body—made up of the atomic vibrations to which the circulation in various portions of the body is reactive—to get a sun tan would not be well for this body; for it would burn tissue before it would tan. That which would be more effective (if the body is insistent that it desires the tan) would be the use of vinegar and olive oil (not vinegar made from acetic acid, or synthetic vinegar, but the use of that made from the apples) combined with coffee made from resteaming or re-vaporing used coffee grounds. The tannin in each of these, and the acids combined, would become very effective. But it will wear off, of course, in a very short time even—if used.   276-7

Cold and Hot Packs

Pack is the name given generally to a variety of applications, whether the treatment uses a wet or dry towel, hot or cold cloth, blankets or sheets—wrapping either a limb or the whole body—or makes a simple application to a small area of the body. Often the word *pack* is used generically or interchangeably with reference to the applied treatments, much as the words *automobile* or *tree* would be used to cover various types or species.

Many types of packs are mentioned in the Cayce readings—from Atomidine to Epsom salts to grape to mullein to turpentine—as well as simple hot and cold packs. It should be noted, however, that the terminology in the Cayce readings is not always exact; for example, the universal term *pack* may be used, as in *grape pack*, when the proper designation is *grape poultice*. Yet the descriptive terms as stated in the readings' excerpts are retained as written, in keeping with quoting the exact wording from the Cayce text.

WHEN TO USE COLD AND WHEN TO USE HEAT

How do you decide whether to apply heat or cold to an injury? Sprains, strains, an aching back, a bump, or a pulled muscle—any soft tissue injury—are all candidates for hot or cold packs.

In general one should apply ice or cold immediately to injuries. Cold helps reduce swelling and pain by restricting blood flow, which in turn slows the inflammatory response. Cold also slows nerve conduction, decreasing the pain caused by the injury. As a general rule, if the area feels warm or inflamed to the touch, apply cold. If it feels cool to the touch, apply heat. Not sure? Use a cold application.

A cold or ice pack is left on for a shorter period of time than a hot pack. Different suggestions for lengths of time have been recommended by different experts, yet the caution is not to overdo the icing—no longer than twenty minutes at a time. Elevate the injured area, as well, to help restrict the swelling and prevent further tissue damage. You may also apply a pressure bandage or splint over the affected area.

Once the swelling has subsided (after approximately forty-eight to seventy-two hours), you may begin the heat application, which stimulates blood flow and loosens stiff muscles. Usually two to three days after an injury and following a cold application, the blood flow has begun to return to normal, decreasing the risk of swelling and internal bleeding. The warmth increases the blood flow, opens the blood vessels, and helps the area to return to a full range of motion. The hot pack, then, is much more effective at this time than a cold treatment.

A large portion of Cayce's references on cold packs actually relates to alternating hot and cold applications, sometimes referred to as "contrast treatments." These treatments will be discussed in the information following "Hot Packs."

With the appropriate applications of heat and cold, your healing process will be enhanced and your recovery time will be reduced.

COLD PACKS

INDICATIONS

Cooling neck and forehead during warm sitz, steam, or hot bath; fever; fresh injury (within 24 to 48 hours after incident); hemorrhaging; inflammation; intestinal problems; muscle spasms; old injury that has been reactivated and reinjured; painful areas

CONTRAINDICATIONS

Already chilled or debilitated, cardiac disorders, diabetes, hypersensitivity to or fear of cold, hypertension, impaired circulation, impaired sensation, Raynaud's disease, use carefully with persons who cannot communicate (such as babies, elderly, or unconscious people)

MATERIALS NEEDED

Towel or cloth—to dip into cold water

Dry towel or piece of plastic—to cover wet towel

Source of cold water: container or bucket of ice cubes to which water has been added

Towel or plastic (optional)—to place under the treated area to protect the sheets

FREQUENCY OF APPLICATION

Apply for 15 minutes every four hours for 2 to 3 days, reapply every half hour for the first 4 to 6 hours (following initial injury), re-dip when cold sensation has diminished, replace frequently (different frequencies given by various sources)

LENGTH OF TIME OF APPLICATION

Less than 1 minute, 1 to 5 minutes, 5 to 8 minutes, 15 to 20 minutes; *no more than 20 minutes at a time*

LOCATION OF APPLICATION

On back of neck and forehead (while in steam cabinet, hot tub, or hot bath), over abdomen, directly on injured or painful area

SIZE OF PACK

Large enough to cover injured or painful area

Washcloth for back of neck and forehead

EXPECTED EFFECTS/PURPOSES

Decreases metabolism, respiratory rate, pulse rate, and blood flow to area

Numbs pain receptors

Lowers core temperature

Slows circulation and digestion

Decreases fever and inflammation

Reduces muscle spasms and swelling

Arrests hemorrhaging

Enhances urine production, muscle tone, thyroid activity, elimination, immune system, and red and white corpuscle production

DIRECTIONS

Place a dry towel or plastic sheet under the area to be iced to protect the underlying sheets or bedding. Determine your source of cold, icy water, such as a bucket or container of ice cubes with enough water added to soak thoroughly a towel or washcloth. Dip the cloth into the container, wring it out, then roll it in a backward and forward motion over the skin to acclimate the body area, gradually slowing down the movements and eventually resting the cold cloth completely onto the skin. Wrap the wet cloth securely and snugly around the injured area, covering the area needing attention. An extra dry towel or a sheet of plastic is placed on top of the wet cloth and tucked in. This helps contain the cold temperature and allows the body heat to warm the cloth more intensely, since one's body—after its initial chilly reaction to the cold—will attempt to warm the area and stabilize the cold temperature.

After a few minutes, when the skin loses the cold sensation, the outermost dry towel and the wet, cold towel are removed. The wet towel is re-dipped in the cold water and placed back onto the skin. Re-cover the area with the dry towel. This procedure may be repeated, with each application lasting no more than twenty minutes at a time. (See *Frequency of Application* and *Length of Time of Application.*)

DIRECTIONS FROM THE READINGS

For a forty-eight-year-old man suffering from gastritis and headaches (reading given on July 5, 1936):

> . . . the applications . . . to the head and to the feet—of something cool;

not cold or ice cold but cool to the head.   261-23

For an adult male with fever, impaired locomotion, and a tendency toward spinal meningitis (reading given on October 30, 1931):

... keep those of ice packs or cold packs at the top of head rather than at the base of the spine ...   5464-1

For an approximately fifty–three–year–old woman with pain in her right knee, as well as varicose veins, hypertension, and tendencies toward neuritis and rheumatism (reading given on August 18, 1931):

... Of mornings we would rub the body along the spine thoroughly with cold rubs. The colder the better, from the base of the head to the end of the spine. If the cloths or towels used as rubs are wrung out of *ice* water, all the better ...   327-2

[Later, in answer to her question about the cause of her itching ears, the reading stated: " ... Increasing the circulation by these cold rubs, we will have this eliminated ... " (327-2)]

For a fifty–one–year–old woman suffering from acidity, asthma tendencies, and hypertension (reading given on July 16, 1942):

Following the colonic, there should be a very mild sweat in the dry cabinet—just sufficient to raise the temperature to a sweat ... (and do keep cold packs on the head, even when the fume bath is given— and watch the pulse with this) ...   2782-1

For an adult male who had been an epileptic for over twenty-five years (reading given on December 9, 1910):
[He was advised to do short, periodic cold applications to his spine, usually on the upper cervicals.]

... The action of the cold along the spine is ... stimulating and has medicinal properties, combined with electrical force {*Violet Ray*}.

34-4

[Slight alterations were made from one reading to the next regarding temperature and length of application, all dependent upon his progress.]

TESTIMONIALS/RESULTS

Mr. [261]'s wife wrote at the end of the year, on December 30, 1936, that her husband:

> " . . . still seems very tired most of the time {*he had been suffering from gastritis and headaches; see* Directions from the Readings} . . . He can't seem to follow your advice entirely and stop worrying and working so hard."   261-27, Report #2

He was in the banking business and obtained several readings combining business information with health advice. After his last reading, his thirty–fifth, he wrote:

> " . . . For some time after receiving the reading I felt considerably better. If I don't now it is only because I don't continue to do all the things the reading recommended. I am so very busy these days that I find it hard to do all the things that I should . . . "   261-35, Report #1

The sister of Mr. [34], a longtime epileptic (see *Directions from the Readings*), wrote that following each reading:

> " . . . a course of treatment was instituted {*cold packs along the spine*}, since which time he has improved wonderfully, and seems to be on the road to ultimate recovery . . . "   34-8, Report #1

The results were astounding:

> " . . . He scarcely, if ever, has any more spells and they are hardly perceptible, while he formerly had quite a number each day, falling any

place he might happen to be, oftentimes sustaining painful injuries. We have ample reasons to believe that through the mystic power of young Mr. Cayce a permanent cure shall be consummated."

34-8, Report #1

In July 1960 Dr. Walter Pahnke added this notation to the readings' supplemental reports:

" . . . There is {a} good possibility that the diagnosis is epilepsy, but the type of epilepsy cannot be definitely established." 34-8, Report #3

ADDITIONAL INFORMATION

In addition to using towels, cloths, or linens dipped in cold water to apply as a pack, another way of using cold compresses is with an ice bag, ice cap, or ice pack. These insulated bags, filled with ice chips or ice cubes, help make the application of very cold temperatures a little easier on the skin. Readily available for use, they are placed directly onto the area of pain or soreness. The softness of the bag's material enables the pack to contour easily to the body area, surrounding the tissue with a comfortable cooling compress.

If you do not have such a pack on hand, a bag of frozen peas, corn, or other frozen vegetable works just as well as the standard ice pack. For such an application, you can place a thin cloth or towel between the bag and your skin to prevent frostbite. If your skin begins to itch or tingle after you apply the pack, remove the pack immediately as it may be a sign of impending frostbite.

Nearly twenty readings mention an ice pack or ice cap, mostly used in traditional ways: to reduce fever, curb inflammation, or as a cold compress on the head during steam baths or warm tub baths. In the latter case, ice packs or cold compresses to keep the head cool are a welcome relief during such a bath where, as the readings often state, the water should be kept " . . . as warm, or as hot as the body can well stand; letting the body remain as long as possible {in the Epsom salts bath} just so as not to weaken it too much." (2768–1) (See also the chapter on "Epsom Salts Bath.") For the steam cabinet, however, the A.R.E. Spa fol-

lows Dr. Harold J. Reilly's directive: remain no longer than twenty minutes in the cabinet; too long a stay depletes the body's minerals and
may dehydrate a person, resulting in fatigue and lightheadedness. (*See
also* the chapter on "Steam/Fume Bath" for more information.) One principle in hydrotherapy is: *less is more.*

HOT PACKS

INDICATIONS
Arthritis (not rheumatoid), bursitis, colds, gout, influenza, joint pain,
muscle aches, neuralgia, preparation for spinal adjustments, sprains, strains

CONTRAINDICATIONS
Acute inflammation, being already overheated or dehydrated, bleeding, burns, cancer, cardiac disorders, diabetes, hypertension, impaired
sensation, Raynaud's disease, use carefully with persons who cannot
communicate (such as babies, elderly, or unconscious people)
Be careful of the range of heat; avoid burning the skin by periodic
checking of the skin; feelings of faintness, dizziness, rapid pulse, and
nausea might indicate a lowering of blood pressure; when muscles become too relaxed, fatigue and lethargy may result

MATERIALS NEEDED
Towel or cloth—to dip into hot water
Dry towel or piece of plastic—to cover wet towel
Source of hot water and container or bucket to which hot water has
been added
Towel or plastic (optional)—to place under the treated area to protect
the sheets
Heating pad or hot water bottle (optional)—to maintain heat

FREQUENCY OF APPLICATION
Depends upon the desired effect, the resultant reaction, and the condition being treated; may change hot towel every 3 to 5 minutes until
20 minutes of duration

LENGTH OF TIME OF APPLICATION

Short: 3 to 5 minutes (stimulating—for muscle fatigue)

Long: 5 to 20 minutes (depressive—decreases circulation and increases metabolism)

LOCATION OF APPLICATION

Place directly on injured or painful area

SIZE OF PACK

Large enough to cover injured or painful area

EXPECTED EFFECTS/PURPOSES

Increases metabolism, respiration, pulse rate, and blood volume

Decreases tissue tone and blood pressure

Decreases peripheral white and red blood cell count

Relaxes nerves and muscles (sedative)

Loosens chest congestion (expectorant)

Relieves pain: decreases nerve sensation (analgesic)

DIRECTIONS

Place a dry towel or plastic sheet under the area to be warmed to protect the underlying sheets or bedding. Determine your source of hot water, such as a hot plate, a bucket, or a container with enough hot water to soak thoroughly a towel or washcloth. Dip the cloth into the container, wring it out, and roll it in a backward and forward motion over the skin to acclimate the body area, gradually slowing down the movements and eventually resting the hot cloth completely onto the skin. Wrap the cloth securely and snugly around the injured area, covering the area needing attention. An extra dry towel or a sheet of plastic is placed on top of the wet cloth and tucked in. This extra towel helps contain the warm temperature. To maintain a steady flow of heat, a hot water bottle or a heating pad may be placed over the plastic sheet or dry towel (the plastic or towel also prevents the heating pad from getting damp).

When the wet towel begins to cool (if no hot water bottle or heating pad is used), it can be removed and re-dipped in the hot water, then placed back on the skin and rewrapped with a dry towel or plastic sheet. This procedure may be followed from three to five minutes (for a short pack) to five to twenty minutes (for a long hot pack), depending upon the condition that is being treated.

DIRECTIONS FROM THE READINGS

For a female adult suffering from spinal lesions (reading given on September 23, 1935):

> We would make changes in these {*lesions*} by adjustments. But before making the adjustments we would apply *wet* heat. This is preferable to dry heat, for it will make for a centralizing of the superficial circulation more about those areas.
>
> So, we would apply heavy wet towels—or packs made with towels that are wet or damp sufficient to draw the heat or the activity of the circulation through the heat at the coccyx (or the lower end of the spine and the sacral area) and from the 5th dorsal to the 2nd and 3rd cervical.
>
> And then make the adjustments. Do this about twice each week.
>
> 1008-1

For a twenty-four-year-old woman with a torn ligament in her left knee due to a skiing accident; surgery was advised by her physician (reading given on May 5, 1942):

> The specific disturbance that we find from the injury in the left limb or knee—where there is a strained ligament, between the upper and lower portion (and this in the right side of same under kneecap)—it would be better *not* to have operative measures, but to apply—daily—in the afternoon or when ready to retire—wet heat; that is, heavy towels wrung out of hot water, as hot as body can well stand. Apply these once or twice and then thoroughly massage the knee, especially around the cap and on the inside and under side, with *salt* that has been well saturated with Pure Apple Vinegar.   1771-4

For a seven-year-old girl whose chief complaint was fever along with physicians' diagnosis of juvenile rheumatism (reading given on November 29, 1943):

> If these areas are still in those positions of being hard to change, relax same throughout the sacral and the coccyx area with wet heat before making corrections, as also the whole cervical area. Apply heavy towels wrung out of hot water, as hot as the body can stand it. Repeat this several times. Lay these on the body, cover with an oilcloth or the like and then let the heat gradually die away. Do this some two to three times, just before the corrections are attempted, and these will be much more easily made.   2883-2

TESTIMONIALS/RESULTS

Answers to a questionnaire on July 21, 1951, written by Mrs. [1771]:

> " . . . From a skiing accident on March 3, 1942, the main ligament in left knee was torn loose. The doctor advised soaking in hot Epsom Salts, which gave no benefit at all; it might have prevented inflammation from getting worse, but certainly did no healing. A week later the doctor advised surgery, that it was all that could be done. That's when I got the reading, 1771-4. {*See* Directions from the Readings.} It worked! Marked improvement within a month, gradually possible to have complete flexibility in knee. Didn't go back to the doctor who was supposed to be the best, after he suggested the operation. That fall I went on trail walks, which were long but not difficult. For about a year I abstained from dancing, bowling, and skating (I never skied again). I've climbed mountains, etc., never had the slightest trouble only early July this year, during a second pregnancy, in walking down steps especially I noticed a pain under the kneecap on the inside of the left leg. I used the oil massage {*formula given in the reading consisted of peanut oil, oil of pine needles and sassafras root, and dissolved lanolin*} and it disappeared."   1771-5, Report #2

Answers to a questionnaire on June 9, 1951, written by the mother of [2883]:

" . . . Chief Complaint: Fever—feet affected. Date of Onset: During the fall of 1942. Duration: Two years, approximately. Reoccurrence: During fall of 1943 . . . Physicians' Diagnosis and Treatment: Juvenile rheumatism . . . {*See* Directions from the Readings.}

" . . . Second Physical {*Reading*}—Hot water packs—three times just before corrections are attempted, special attention to sacral and coccyx area—coordinate with 3rd cervical area. Duration of Treatment: No. of years: 2 . . . Results of Treatment: Cured . . .

" . . . On doctor's advice, patient was kept out of school for ten weeks during first attack, and nine weeks when the second attack occurred. Long rest periods each day were deemed advisable; patient was allowed up and around the house in between rest periods and could take short rides in the car.

"Patient was taken back to Dr. { . . . } after second reading and he followed through with the treatments."   2883-2, Report #1

Follow-up note from a friend of the girl's mother over a month after her first reading: " . . . {*the doctor*} seems to have discharged [2883] as completely taken care of as far as his treatments are concerned. Her mother is delighted over the quick results from following the reading and the child has been back in school for two weeks now . . . " (2883-1, Report #1) The mother later confirmed that her daughter was apparently well.

Some years later the mother's friend again wrote:

" . . . [2883] is a fine looking, attractive, capable girl, in second year high school, a credit to anyone for intelligence, appearance, etc. No sign of any physical disturbance from the trouble she had as a small child when the reading was had, and no repetition during her childhood."   2883-2, Report #2

ALTERNATING HOT AND COLD

Sometimes referred to as "contrast treatments," alternating hot and cold packs (when neither temperature is contraindicated) can be a rather powerful, effective application, utilizing the beneficial effects of both temperatures. The process is described by author Maureen O'Rourke: "Heat application will bring fresh, oxygenated blood to the area to begin healing and carry out toxic waste products and debris. It is followed by the cold influence, which will limit pain and swelling, while it slows the metabolism, which causes the buildup of waste products. Swift healing and pain relief are the most obvious results of this powerful contrast effect . . . " (*Hydrotherapy and Heliotherapy*, p. 18)

Various Cayce suggestions for packs relate to this hot/cold alternation. Usually one begins with a hot pack, switching to cold, then back and forth, ending with a cold pack. The hot packs are left on for a longer time than the cold packs, keeping within the *Length of Time of Application* guidelines listed under **Cold Packs** and **Hot Packs**. O'Rourke offers an example of how this sequence could work: " . . . an effective recipe is 3 minutes of hot water immersion, followed by 30 seconds to 1 minute of cold application. Begin with heat and end with cold, repeating the sequence 6 to 8 times, allowing approximately ½ hour for the whole treatment." (p. 18) After the final cold application, the skin is patted dry. If needed, some warmth may be restored to the individual—such as taking a warm foot bath, covering oneself with a warm blanket, or any other way to warm up.

A representation of this application, therefore, would consist of:

(1)   beginning with heat: 3 minutes
(2)   adding the cold: 30 seconds to 1 minute
(3)   repeating 6 to 8 times; total time: ½ hour
(4)   ending with cold application
(5)   patting the skin dry
(6)   warming the person, if needed

Applications may also be mixed (without using packs), such as using a heating pad, alternating it with ice massage; soaking in a bath of alternating hot and cold water; or taking a hot shower followed by a cool rinse.

The indications and contraindications for heat and cold apply to these contrast treatments as well. Following is some additional information from the Cayce readings on the use of alternating hot and cold packs.

INDICATIONS, LOCATION, LENGTH OF TIME OF APPLICATION, AND FREQUENCY:

Baldness: packs on scalp, face muscles, throat, neck, and head; once a week (935-1)

Cholecystitis (inflammation of gallbladder): packs on abdomen and lower stomach area; 1½ to 2 hours daily (1826-1)

Facial tic: packs on neck and between shoulders; 15 minutes every other day after osteopathic treatments (1434-3)

Infertility: packs over appendix and right groin area (where distress was located) at least twice a week for 2 to 3 hours; about 20 minutes for each pack; rest afterwards (349-20)

Impaired locomotion: packs on lumbar and 9th dorsal area especially, along with adjustments; 2 to 3 times a week for 5 weeks (2507-1)

Nervous system incoordination (woman had weak feet and arches with occasional falls): packs along the cerebrospinal system " . . . with special reference being given to the sacral and lumbar axis . . . "; spinal adjustments done before packs; frequency and length of time determined by the hydrotherapist (2394-1)

Psoriasis-like lesions: packs placed on skin lesions; a few minutes for each (982-1)

Sluggish or slow eliminations: packs " . . . to produce a greater reaction . . . "; area not specified (337-24)

Toxemia: packs on abdomen; every other day for 3 weeks, then once a week (1938-1)

DIRECTIONS FROM THE READINGS

For a forty-seven-year-old man suffering from a " . . . nervous tension which of course brings headaches and indigestion . . . " (877-28, Background #2) and dermatitis (reading given on February 2, 1939):

(Q) What about the nervous conditions?
(A) These show a great deal of improvement . . . when the hydrotherapy treatments are given we would have the general massage, the sweats, or the hot and cold water with the massage . . . The hot and cold hydrotherapy treatment—that is, hot water, cold water; hot compresses, cold

compresses. These alternated will aid the nervous system.   877-28

For an eighteen-year-old woman suffering from a facial tic which caused twitching in her eye, mouth, and tongue (reading given on December 23, 1938):

> ... when the hot and cold packs are applied, make them alternately; applying them from about the neck to that area between and below the shoulders; as hot as the body can stand, and then just as cold as it can stand. One right after the other, for fifteen minutes; changing them at least eight times during such a fifteen minute period. This would be done *after* the osteopathic treatment, every other day, you see. 1434-3

For a forty-eight-year-old woman suffering from cholecystitis (inflammation of the gallbladder) (reading given on February 20, 1939):

> ... we would begin the use of Hot and Cold Packs over the abdominal and lower stomach area; especially the liver. These would be given alternately, you see, for a few hours every day—when they are begun—for a few days. In this manner they would be the more effective, or give them at least for an hour and a half to two hours each day, changing them every few minutes—first the hot, then the cold.   1826-1

For a thirty-five-year-old woman with a sluggish liver and abdomen and who was trying to get pregnant (reading given on July 6, 1939):

> We would apply at least twice each week the hot and cold packs, about two or three times each, first hot and then cold, for about twenty minutes each, over this area {*lower right groin or lower abdomen*}; but not at or close to the menstrual period, see? Two or three applications of the hot, two or three of the cold, you see; one right after the other. Then afterwards the body should rest well, after such have been used.
> 349-20

For a twenty-four-year-old man with circulatory disturbances (incoordination), dermatitis, and occasional chest pains (reading given on February 18, 1939):

> These {*"disturbances in the circulatory forces of the body—as is indicated in the irritation to those superficial portions of the body"*} as we find would be best reduced by the use, about an hour each evening, of the hot and cold packs alternately—very hot, very cold, see? Let these applications last about an hour or the like, changing the packs about every five to ten minutes—using first hot, then cold.   1528-3

(Notice that the reading does not state where to place the packs; evidently it is where "irritation" has appeared on the skin, such as dermatitis. The next paragraph in the reading advises Mr. [1528] to bathe his "hands in a weak solution of Atomidine water," so this might be the targeted area for the packs.)

Electric Vibrator

Varieties of electric vibrators are available on the market today and come in handy to help with easing tense muscles, increasing blood circulation, and promoting a restful sleep. Over 270 readings mention this hand-held appliance, sometimes described as an electrically driven vibrator or electric device, and it is recommended in many types of cases.

The attachments most often mentioned by Cayce include the sponge, suction, cup, or hard (knob end). It can be used as an adjunct to massage or spinal manipulations, and should be placed directly on the skin, not over the clothing.

INDICATIONS

Backache, baldness, dizziness, headaches, hoarseness, insomnia, leg pain, lung congestion, muscle contractions, nerve exhaustion, overtaxation, poor eyesight, possession, restlessness, shortness of breath, spinal subluxations, throat and head congestion, toxemia

CONTRAINDICATIONS

Do not use the same day that you are taking Al-Caroid, an antacid compound (690-1)

MATERIALS NEEDED

Electric vibrator
Several types of attachments (included with purchase of the device)

FREQUENCY OF APPLICATION

Daily; every other day; 1, 2, 3, or 4 times a week; series: 6 to 8 days, rest for 2 or 3 days, resume; 10 to 20 days, rest for a period, then resume

WHEN TO USE THE ELECTRIC VIBRATOR

Evenings before retiring, mornings, when massages are impractical, " . . . when the body needs it for rest . . . " (4168-1), when there is heaviness in the feet and lower limbs, when " . . . the body is trembly or gets excited easily . . . " (303-20), prior to or after a massage, after crude oil treatment on the scalp

LENGTH OF TIME OF APPLICATION

A few minutes, 3 to 5 minutes, 5 to 15 minutes, 15 to 30 minutes, more than 30 minutes, 35 to 50 minutes

LOCATION OF APPLICATION

Abdomen, above diaphragm area, across lumbar area, across the hips, across the shoulders, arms, each side of spine, face, head, hip joint, lower extremities down to the toes, lower limbs on the sciatic nerves, neck, scalp, whole length of spine

EXPECTED EFFECTS/PURPOSES

Relaxes congestion along the spine
Eases muscular contraction
Promotes a restful sleep
Adds energy to the blood and nerves
Helps destroy foreign matter in the system

Stimulates superficial circulation and centers along the cerebrospinal system

Relieves tension

Helps " . . . in the general eliminations." (303–41)

Increases " . . . circulation to the sensory forces . . . " (404–6)

Rejuvenates the nerve centers

Aids in distributing the oil from massages

DIRECTIONS

Easy-to-follow directions are usually included with the purchase of an electric vibrator. Illustrations and photos may also help to explain the workings of the device and how it is used. Additionally the Cayce readings offer guidelines for its particular application in accordance with the individual's specific need, mentioning as well the proper applicator to use. (See *Directions from the Readings.*)

Several people asked for clarification on the device itself; for example, " . . . what kind of an electric vibrator would be used . . . ?" and the reply was: "That with which we give the electric massage, those electrically driven . . . " (1112–1)

Another asked, "Is that the machine that fits over the hand as used by {a} masseur?" Cayce answered: "This may be used, but the electric driven machine is better for this particular body." (140–35)

One person wondered if the electric vibrator were strong enough, and Cayce replied: "This does very good. These vibrations from this will be better than vibratory forces . . . " (195–15)

This hand–held appliance conveys a vibratory effect wherever it is placed on the body. After being plugged in, the machine, guided manually over the skin—not over the clothing—helps to break up congestion, ease muscle tension, and increase circulation, bringing an overall relaxing and soothing effect to the body. Cayce told one person to " . . . add energy to blood, to nerve, by adding electrical forces, or vibration as may be attained by the body through the electric vibrator . . . " (4785–1) In several instances, the readings describe the vibrations as "deep" and " . . . preferable even to adjustments *or* manipulations . . . " (404–6) In one case during the period of rest from the vibrator the person was to receive an osteopathic manipulation or a massage.

Several readings point out the uses of particular applicators; for instance, the cup or suction applied to the scalp after a massage with crude oil and white Vaseline (for baldness). Another individual was told to use the cup alongside the spine:

> . . . Rather than using this sliding it up and down, use it in a suction manner; that is, raise it and press down—very close, of course—all along the spine. Raise it gently so that the cup creates a suction. And this should be used with the body almost bare, or a very thin cloth between the body and the appliance.   313-8

For tight muscles the vibrator with the ball applicator can be used in conjunction with heat:

> We would use more of the heat applications, and a deep vibration with the ball or the harder applicator of the electrically driven vibrator—especially so in the lower lumbar area and in the portion of the hip joint where there is the muscular contraction.   348-20

One woman was told: " . . . Use the sponge applicator about the face, head and neck, and especially over the antrum, back of the head, the throat and the neck. Use the cup applicator along the cerebrospinal system and the upper portion of the body, across the diaphragm . . . " (2309-1) The vibrator would not only produce better rest, but it would also stimulate the superficial circulation.

The electric vibrator, then, provides a mechanical way of relaxing the body and inducing better health and balance to the system.

DIRECTIONS FROM THE READINGS

For a fifty-nine-year-old man with incoordinations in circulation, assimilation, and elimination (reading given on December 15, 1937):

> (Q) What can be done to relieve terrible headaches all along?
> (A) These arise as much from the digestive forces as from any other

thing, and as we find with the change of the diet and the use of the vibrator as indicated, electrically driven, you see—using the cup, especially above the diaphragm area or throughout the whole the cup would be better (the cup applicator, you see), or as to produce a percussion or suction or drawing—given just before retiring—these would make for the inclinations for the body to rest better, and relieve the headaches.   389-9

For a fourteen–year–old girl with abdominal adhesions and incoordination of the nervous system and glands (reading given on January 4, 1935):

(Q) What is to be done to enable the body to fall asleep at night?
(A) The use of the electrically driven vibrator should make for the relaxing sufficiently for the body to fall to sleep. Use this over the cerebrospinal system, or around the back of the head, the neck, across the shoulders, even down to the lower portion of the body, as has been indicated.   728-2

A fifty–six–year–old woman, with poor eliminations and nervous system incoordination, felt that a "power" had taken possession over her (reading given on April 18, 1938):

Every day, preferably in the evening, use the Electrically Driven Vibrator across the lower portion of the cerebrospinal system, from the base of the brain to the end of the spine. Use the applicator that forms a suction upon the body itself; that is, the cup applicator. Then, use it across the abdomen; following the line of the colon, from the liver area down to the caecum, or opposite the right hip bone, then up and across the abdomen just below the navel and then down to the left side opposite the left hip bone. If these instructions are followed, it will require about fifteen to eighteen to twenty minutes. Don't just run the vibrator over those areas, but take time to give a thorough treatment. Come down, you see, along the cerebrospinal system—that's along the backbone, on either side of the backbone, and especially across the lower

portion of the *pelvis* area—that's across the small of the back and to
the end of the spine! *Come down* the spine, you see, with the strokes;
not just running the machine back and forth! Then use it across the
abdomen, coming down from the liver area on the right side to the
caecum, or that area just below or opposite the right hip bone. Then up
just a little farther, you see, to the left; to that area directly below the
navel area but on the right side. Then cross under the navel to the left
portion of the colon. This is following, of course, the course of the colon.   1572-1

For a sixty-five-year-old woman suffering from toxemia and spinal
subluxations (reading given on February 21, 1941):

Two, three to four times a week we would use at home the Electrically
Driven Vibrator; which would necessarily be given by someone else in
the home, you see. Do not give this merely as something just to be
gotten through with, but slowly, persistently, for at least thirty-five to
fifty minutes; along the cerebrospinal system, along the limbs, and especially over the area of the 9th dorsal and lumbar axis. Use the Cup
Applicator. Afterwards give the body a hand massage using the equal
combination of the Olive Oil and Peanut Oil.   464-31

TESTIMONIALS/RESULTS

Mr. [5291], a fifty-year-old man, had a health reading on June 27,
1944. He was suffering from a leakage of the heart, seborrheic dermatitis, and cholecystalgia (biliary colic)—all of which were cured. On September 9, 1946, he wrote: " . . . I am enjoying good health after following
the instructions given in my reading." (5291-1, Report #2) Later, on January 8, 1947, in answer to an inquiry he replied in more detail:

"My chief complaint was a pain in right side of abdomen, under short
ribs, for six months prior to the reading. I had an attack several years
previous—whole nervous system was affected. I was steadily getting
worse until {*I followed*} the treatments as directed in the reading,
though I was still able to work. I started taking treatments from Dr.

[...], a mechanotherapist, after receiving the reading. I took two treatments three days apart before I gave him the reading. He asked where I got it and how. I told him and gave him *There Is a River* to read. (Several people here have read the book, among them four doctors, medical, osteopath, and chiropractor.) I used the Castor Oil Packs, the prescribed diet, the high colonic irrigations, and the electrically driven vibrator over a three-month period. Relief was marked. I have had no recurrence of the symptoms."   5291-1, Report #3

In a letter written on May 11, 1926, Mrs. [1187], a forty-seven year old suffering from toxemia and spinal subluxations, described how much she had been helped by her reading and would have been helped more if she'd gotten the electric vibrator sooner.

" . . . I am using it now and have had such restful nights since I first began using it."   1187-4, Report #1

The husband of [483] (no age given) wrote to Cayce on March 13, 1934, two months after his wife's reading, describing the attempts he was making to apply the suggestions recommended, while needing to modify some of the treatments based on his wife's response. She had neurasthenia (weakness of the nervous system) and had some difficulty with the applications:

" . . . The electric vibrator has not been used so faithfully. She seems unable to stand it on the head, even with very light pressure though we have used it on the head several times. The vibrator over upper spine and base of brain seems to give some headache and nausea so we have only given treatment then every alternate day . . . "   483-1, Report #9

Several paragraphs later he wrote: " . . . I have been unable financially to have an expert use the vibrator and Violet Ray and have used them on her myself. I have used them as nearly the instructions as I know . . . " (483-1, Report #9) He asked for some clarification on modifying the instructions and continued to work sporadically with her condition. A month later she had a check reading, which noted her hypo-chondria. Several months later Cayce learned that Mrs. [483] had been admitted to a state hospital and was released some months later. Her husband feared that she would have to return. No further information is available.

ADDITIONAL INFORMATION

Frequently in the readings, the placement of the electric vibrator is alongside the spine (that is, on either side of the spine), and usually the device is to be applied along the spine's *entire length*. The reason for this position was mentioned in several readings:

For "intense pain in the head" one woman was advised to use the appliance at " . . . the eighth, ninth and tenth dorsals {*thoracic*}, the fifth and sixth dorsals and the third and fourth cervicals. This we will find will relax the muscular forces along these regions where the contraction begins in the nerve forces here . . . " (3964-1) She would also obtain a more restful sleep.

Another woman was advised to use the vibrator " . . . from the 4th dorsal to the 6th and 7th dorsal; preferably along either *side* of the cerebro-spinal column, rather than directly over the area . . . so that the connections here, between the cerebro-spinal system and the sympathetic nervous system, receive those impulses through the creation of a gathering of the circulation. This will tend to make for the releasing of those tensions, and thus make for food values and food activities to be less severe upon this portion of the digestive system." (404-6)

Later in her reading she asked a question about improving her eyesight and was told:

> Eyesight will improve; for this, as indicated, is from the very nature of the applications to the deeper cerebrospinal system—or for the deeper circulation, by the application of the electrically driven vibration . . . for the *vibrations* reach to various portions of not only ganglia but the bursae along the flow of the nerve forces of the system . . . for the nerve ends of the sensory force (eyes, ears, taste, hearing) reach to the upper portion of the dorsal area, or the 3rd, 4th and 5th dorsal center.

> These are a portion of that to be covered by the applications as indicated, and will be helpful in this direction . . .   404-6

One final excerpt again mentions the purpose for this particular placement alongside the spine: coordination of the two nervous systems, as well as promoting rest for the body:

> . . . have the electrically driven vibrator along the whole length of the cerebro-spinal system—that the body may rest the better, that the body may have the better reactions from the organs of the body following same . . . that the whole of the system may receive those impetuses from the exercising of the ganglia along the cerebro-spinal system, as to make for a better coordination with the sympathetic and cerebro-spinal system, and a stimul{*us*} from the ganglia especially in the upper cervical, or 3rd and 4th cervical, the 3rd and 4th dorsal, or the brachial center, and those of the lumbar—in the 3rd and 4th lumbar, that the whole of the body may *rest* the much easier.   578-1

Electric vibrators are readily available in most pharmacies or in the medicine section of many grocery stores. They are relatively easy to use and provide relaxation, stimulation, and relief for one's body.

Epsom Salts Bath

In our fast-paced world taking a bath in a tub may seem indulgent or time-consuming. Yet many people today do enjoy the pure pleasure of luxuriating in a warm bath or hot tub. Bathing therapy, known as balneology or balneotherapy, though ancient in origin, is an accepted form of medical treatment throughout Europe and other parts of the world as well. When we place a substance such as Epsom salts into the water, we can increase the bath's potency and thus enhance the benefits.

Epsom salts, which is hydrated magnesium sulfate ($MgSO_4 \cdot 7H_2O$), is a one-hundred-percent natural mineral that, added to a tub of warm water, can provide soothing relief to one's body. A member of the salt family, it gets its name from a city in southern England, Epsom, where the salts were originally obtained from the water of a mineral spring there.

In the Cayce readings, the use of Epsom salts is mentioned over eight hundred times and is recommended in a variety of ways. One hundred individuals were advised to use it as a bath, most often in conjunction with massages, colonics, the Wet-Cell Appliance, and/or dosages of Atomidine.

The amount of salt crystals to be used varies widely as well as the gallon content of the tub. On the carton's label is noted the manufacturer's recommendation: two cups of salt per one gallon of warm water. A three-pound box of Epsom salts contains six cups.

Most modern bathtubs hold about twenty gallons of water; the larger, older tubs may hold about thirty. For nearly half of the individuals advised in the readings to take an Epsom salts bath, the salt-and-water content amounted to a "saturated solution"; that is, enough salt is added to the warm water so that the maximum amount is dissolved, eventually reaching a point where undissolved crystals remain in the solution.

Since our largest organ, the skin, absorbs liquids and medications (as in dermal patches), it seems likely that it could and would absorb minerals found in the water. In its attempt to balance the percentages of saline content between the solution and the body fluids beneath the skin, the Epsom salts will draw out toxins from the body, inducing perspiration and allowing other naturally occurring minerals to filter into the skin. These minerals, then, are picked up by the blood and intercellular fluids and carried throughout the body, affecting our entire organism.

INDICATIONS

Aches, arthritis, at beginning of cold and flu symptoms, bruises, catarrh, circulation, fatigue, glandular disturbances, headaches, impaired locomotion, incoordination, injuries, lesions, lumbago, muscle stiffness and pain, neuritis, paralysis, prolapsis, rheumatism and rheumatic tendencies, sciatica, scleroderma, sore joints, sprains, toxemia, venereal disease (aftereffects)

CONTRAINDICATIONS

Cardiovascular problems, diabetes, high blood pressure, kidney problems—consult with physician before attempting the bath, cuts, lymphedema, open wounds or sores, pregnancy, skin rashes, too debilitated or exhausted, not to be used on same day as taking Atomidine, use care with elderly people, may cause dizziness or feeling of fainting—make sure someone is close by to check on or monitor you

MATERIALS NEEDED

Carton of Epsom salts crystals

Bathtub of warm to hot water; *ratio of amount of water to pounds of salt, as given in the Cayce readings:* 10 to 20 gallons of water: 1 or 5 pounds of salt; 15 gallons: 10 lbs.; 20 gallons: 3 to 5 or 10 lbs.; 20 or 25 gallons: 5 to 8, 6 to 10, or 10 to 15 lbs.; 20 to 30 gallons: 1 to 1½, 4 to 5, or 10 to 15 lbs.; 25 gallons: 3 to 5 or 5 to 10 lbs.; 25, 30, 40, or 50 gallons: 5 to 6 or 10 to 15 lbs.; 30 gallons: 20 lbs.; 30, 35, or 40 gallons: 10, 15, or 20 to 25 lbs.; 40 gallons: 10, 12, 15, 20, or 30 lbs.; 40 to 50 gallons: 10 or 20 lbs.; 50 gallons: 10 to 12, 12½, 15, 20, or 25 lbs.; ½ tub of water: 10 lbs.; full tub of water: 5 to 10, 10 to 15, or 20 lbs.; " . . . cover as much of the body as possible . . . " (4293-1): 3 to 5, 5 to 10, 10 to 15, or 20 lbs.

Bath towel to dry off after bathing

Ice pack or cold cloth as compress for head

Cup of cold water for drinking

FREQUENCY OF APPLICATION

Varies depending upon condition treated; daily, weekly, monthly; 5 to 10 days apart, or once or twice weekly (in conjunction with Atomidine) until the condition is improved

LENGTH OF TIME OF APPLICATION

According to one's endurance—from 10 minutes up to 45 minutes or an hour; *warning:* do not overdo, overtax, or weaken the body too much (see also *Contraindications*)

LOCATION OF APPLICATION

Except for the head, the entire body is immersed in warm water that contains a "saturated solution" of Epsom salts (*see* introductory information)

EXPECTED EFFECTS/PURPOSES

Removes lactic acid (built up in muscles after vigorous exercise or strenuous physical activity)

Reduces inflammation

Relieves pain
Promotes relaxation
Induces perspiration
Increases metabolism, heart rate, and body temperature
Detoxifies

DIRECTIONS

The temperature of the bath water is to be as warm as you can tolerate; the water should eventually be deep enough to completely cover
your body, up to your neck. When you are in the tub, you may add hot
water gradually to finish filling the tub, raising the temperature, or you
may simply soak in the full hot tub until the water eventually cools
down. Of course, you may add additional hot water anytime you feel a
decrease in the water temperature, provided there is enough room in
the tub to prevent overflow.

Dr. Harold Reilly, the physiotherapist who followed the Cayce readings and treated people accordingly, advised his clients to begin the
bath with 6 to 8 inches of water (15 to 20 cm) at 102°F (38.9°C)—a pool
thermometer may be used to check the temperature—adding the Epsom salts along with the hot water and stirring often to dissolve the
crystals on the tub bottom. Lie in the tub, gradually adding hotter water
and raising the temperature, reaching from 106° to 108°F (41° to 42°C).
After soaking a while and when you are ready to get out, you may,
according to some instructions, unplug the drain and slowly add cold
water for a gradual, cooling-down effect.

While you are soaking in the tub, the Cayce readings suggest massaging your limbs and torso—or having someone else perform the massage—usually during the entire time of the soak. Often specific areas to
be massaged were described.

In addition, you may place a cold cloth or ice pack on your head to
keep it cool. Several readings such as this one also suggest " . . . keeping
. . . plenty of cold water for the body to drink . . . " while in the tub.
(3244-1)

After your soak, get up slowly and carefully from the tub to dry off,
as you may feel weak or faint. Some readings recommend a sponging

off, a brisk rubdown with a towel, and/or a shower—at times followed by another massage (oils and formulas were specified). The massage may conclude with a grain alcohol rubdown followed by a rest period. Often the baths were advised to be taken in the evenings, so one could afterward go to bed for the night.

At the A.R.E. Health Center and Spa, the client soaks in the tub for twenty minutes, dries off, puts the robe and slippers back on; and, covered with a sheet and towels, rests on the massage table for the remainder of the hour-long appointment, continuing to sweat. Following the rest period ensues a tepid shower to cleanse off the salt water. A massage may follow if the client has requested one.

DIRECTIONS FROM THE READINGS

For a twenty-three-year-old woman with swollen neck glands and tight jaw muscles (reading given on June 19, 1936):

> . . . in *that* evening take an Epsom Salts Bath, as hot as the body can stand. Put at least *ten pounds* of Epsom Salts to forty gallons of water. This should not be too hot when the body first enters same; a little above the temperature of the body. As the body rests in same, gradually add the warmer water. Remain in same for at least thirty minutes to an hour. This will weaken the body somewhat. When the body is sponged off, do not apply *rub* alcohol but equal portion of pure *grain* alcohol and olive oil. Shake them together. Massage them thoroughly into the body from the upper portion of the neck to the tips of the toes; from the shoulders to the tips of the fingers, that the body may absorb these, to produce that reaction of stimulation. *Then* rest from this for two days.
>
> 1058-2

For a forty-seven-year-old woman suffering from arthritis (reading given on January 7, 1938):

> First, begin with Epsom Salts Baths. There should be sufficient water in the bath tub to cover the body, and added to same at least ten to fifteen pounds of Epsom Salts. Let the body lie in this as long as it can,

or for at least twenty to thirty minutes; adding hot water to make it act upon the system. Drink plenty of cold water while in the bath. Take care when coming out of the bath that the body is thoroughly rubbed down, especially the lumbar areas and the limbs and the arms—not merely dried off but thoroughly rubbed; with equal combination of Olive Oil and Peanut Oil. {*Then followed a regimen of alternating doses of Atomidine with the baths; not to be taken on the same days, however.*}

. . . After each of these {*baths*} have a thorough rubdown and let the body be wrapped in {*a*} blanket for at least half an hour to an hour before attempting to move about much.   1514-1

For a forty–four–year–old man who had been " . . . suffering about twelve months {*with*} what the doctors call arthritis, but they can't find out what to do for it . . . " (Report #1); pain in the knee, legs, and arms; and neuritis in shoulder (reading given on June 24, 1942):

Begin with the Epsom Salts Bath at least once each week. Put the body in at least forty gallons of water, in which there would be dissolved at least fifteen to twenty pounds of Epsom Salts. Let this be as hot as the body can stand same, and let the body remain in the tub at least twenty, twenty-five, thirty to thirty-five minutes—if the body can stand it that long. Keep the head cool, by even cold water or ice packs or bags on the head. But while the body is in the bath, do massage ankles, knees and hands (and keep these in the water, or covered with the water). Keep the water as warm, or as hot as the body can well stand; letting the body remain as long as possible just so as not to weaken it too much.

2768-1

For an approximately fifty–year–old (?) woman suffering from headaches and toxemia (reading given on November 15, 1930):

In the beginning, then, we would have those—at least twice each week—of the Epsom Salts baths; that is, three to five pounds to twenty gallons of water, as hot as the body can stand. This to be bathed in, sit

in, lie in, until this has become a cool or cold bath—then be rinsed off
with the tepid water and a thorough rub down the spine . . .   5716-1

TESTIMONIALS/RESULTS

Report from A.R.E. member Mrs. O.J. Lacey in Farmington, Missouri,
in a letter dated January 8, 1966:

> "My doctor approved the Atomidine and salts baths with the peanut oil
> rubs (as recommended in your Circulating Loan File of arthritis cases).
> That was two months ago and my joints are working better than they
> have for several winters."   5361-1, Report #3

From a letter dated April 18, 1972, Mrs. Thomas Hannan of Saint–
Laurent, Quebec, Canada, wrote:

> "You will be happy to know that I am just about cured of arthritis as a
> result of treatment according to the Cayce file. Hospital x-rays con-
> firmed that my whole spine was arthritic in May 1970. I was becoming
> quite crippled and was limited in the use of my arms and legs. I couldn't
> turn in bed nor could I get out of bed without help. Doctors were not at
> all encouraging. I threw away the medication I was using and began
> taking the Atomidine and Epsom salts baths accordingly. {*She also fol-
> lowed the diet and received massages.*} I had amazing results very soon
> and today I am just about back to normal. However, I am still sticking
> with the formula . . . "   5361-1, Report #4

OTHER USES FOR EPSOM SALTS

In the Cayce readings Epsom salts, as noted earlier, are mentioned
over eight hundred times for a variety of uses: as a pack, for a fume
bath, in a tub or sitz bath, or to be taken internally as a laxative. For
further information on these uses, see the chapters on "Epsom Salts
Pack," "Steam/Fume Bath," and "Sitz Bath."

Epsom Salts Pack

A pack is any cloth, towel, or even a sheet or blanket that is used to treat a limb, a part of a limb, or the entire body. The towels may be wet or dry, hot or cold; in the case of Epsom salts packs, the cloth is as hot as one can tolerate.

To assist others in following the suggestions in their readings, Gladys Davis often enclosed directions for certain recommended treatments. Here is one example from a reading for a sixty–five–year–old woman describing how to make an Epsom salts pack:

> " . . . Dissolve as much Epsom Salts as possible in enough water to thoroughly saturate a crash towel. Apply this as hot as possible to the parts affected (where the pain is, when treating yourself; and on the spine where adjustments are needed, when applied by the osteopath). Cover with a dry crash towel to hold the heat. Let it remain until cool. If not entirely {*eased*}, apply again. The Epsom Salts water may be re-heated, but be sure to have as much Epsom Salts in the water as will dissolve each time . . . " 492-1, Report #1

A crash towel, mentioned several times in the previous descrip-

tion, is any coarse cotton or linen cloth with a plain loose weave, usually used for towels, curtains, or clothes.

Sometimes an Epsom salts bath for the entire body was recommended; at other times using only a cloth dipped in Epsom salts and
applied to certain areas of the body was suggested. For several individuals the choice was left up to them which treatment to carry out. The
index to the readings lists over 130 recipients of Epsom salts pack treatments.

Directly treating the affected areas through applying a saturated solution of hot salt greatly reduces the buildup of the body's waste products in tendons, joints, and tissues. The salt draws moisture to itself.
When applied to the body's surface, it causes the internal fluids to move
into circulation, allowing for the drosses, impurities, toxins, and sometimes infected material to make their way out of the body through the
normal channels of elimination, such as sweating. The effects of this
internal cleansing can be noticed by the individual, who might feel a
bit worse after beginning the treatments before he or she begins to feel
better.

After the pack, a gentle peanut oil massage was usually recommended, the oil being applied especially to the affected area or areas
and the massage lasting from fifteen to twenty minutes.

INDICATIONS

Adhesions, arthritis, childbirth (aftereffects), colitis, digestion and
elimination problems, enteritis, feet, fistulas (womb, vagina), flu, gastritis, hemorrhoids, impaired locomotion, infections, injuries, intestinal
problems, kidneys, lesions, liver, lumbago, muscle aches, neuralgia, neuritis, numbness in fingers and toes, painful areas, paralysis, pelvic disorders, prior to menstrual period, rheumatism, sarcoma, sciatica, sinusitis,
spinal subluxations (20 to 30 minutes before adjustments), tic douloureux, to soften hard areas, toxemia, tumors, uremia, uterus, Wilms'
tumor

CONTRAINDICATIONS

Acute, severe inflammation; check for heat sensitivity; impaired sensation; no open wounds, cuts, or sores in area of the pack; use carefully with persons who cannot communicate (such as babies, elderly, or unconscious people)

MATERIALS NEEDED

Epsom salts—about a pound, enough to make a saturated solution

Small basin, tub, pot, or pan in which to dissolve the Epsom salts in hot water

Bath towel, heavy cloth, or linen—to soak in Epsom salted water

Dry towel—to cover wet towel

Hot water—for soaking the towel and dissolving the Epsom salts

Heating pad (optional)—to maintain the heat

Plastic (optional)—to place between the pack and heating pad

Towel or plastic (optional)—to place under the treated area to protect the sheets

FREQUENCY OF APPLICATION

Change when cooled; change when packs harden (become crystallized); change twice; change every ½ hour for 2 to 3 hours; change 3 or 4 times; 3 times each evening; each evening before retiring; daily; every other day; twice a day; once, twice, or 3 times a week; only one application; 3 days in a row; until there is relief

LENGTH OF TIME OF APPLICATION

About 1 hour; once a day 20 to 30 minutes; 45 minutes; once, then reapply in 2 or 3 hours; ½ to ¾ of an hour, leave off for same amount of time, then reapply; once a day for 2 to 3 days; 1 to 1½ hours once a day for 3 days; 2-week period; 12 to 15 days; 3 times a week for 1 week; until it dries on the body

LOCATION OF APPLICATION

Across kidneys; along the spine (before manipulations); areas of severe pain; between shoulders; brachial area (6th and 7th cervical to 7th and 8th dorsal); cecum area; calf of leg; congested areas; directly to muscle contraction and where it originates; fingers; kidney area (small of the back); limbs; lower portion of abdomen; lumbar and sacral areas; solar plexus area (on spine); opposite the affected area; over liver area; " . . . over those plexus and areas from which each of the extremities receive their impulse from the cerebrospinal system . . . " (646-3) [for example, for the hands—place one pack on the 7th and 8th cervical plexus and from the 1st, 2nd, 3rd, and 4th dorsal plexus; "for the lower portions of the body"—place one pack on lumbar area of spine]; painful areas or joints (knees, arms, hands, feet, ankles, hips, shoulders); " . . . where the stiffness or soreness is most pronounced . . . " (1698-1); wrist

SIZE OF PACK
Large enough to cover injured or painful area

EXPECTED EFFECTS/PURPOSES
Reduces and prevents inflammation
Relieves pain and congestion
Relaxes the body system
Eases cramping
Stimulates activity between the upper and lower hepatic circulation
Relieves pressure on bladder and across lumbar/sacral area
Breaks up lesions and accumulations
Enhances bowel movement
Helps to rid the body of toxins
Aids " . . . in setting up better lymph circulation." (623-4)
Increases eliminations
Reduces swelling

DIRECTIONS
To make a saturated solution of Epsom salts with enough water to thoroughly soak a cloth or towel, place very warm or hot water in a basin or tub and gradually add some Epsom salt crystals. Stir the water in order to get as much of the salt to dissolve as possible. Be mindful of the temperature of the water so as not to burn or injure your hands. Also be aware that you may need to increase the heat of the water later since the addition of the crystals may tend to cool the water somewhat.

After stirring the water for a while and adding the crystals, notice if the crystals cease dissolving: that is when you have a saturated solution of Epsom salts. Dip the towel into the hot water, wring it out, and place it directly on the area that needs it. Because of differences in heat tolerance, roll the towel onto the skin, gradually acclimating the skin to the warm temperature. Then place the towel fully onto the area, cover with a large dry towel to enclose the heat, and wait until the body heat cools the area or dries out the towel. Or place a sheet of plastic over the wet towel and put a heating pad turned to "high" over it. Reapply if there is still discomfort or pain. If you reapply, you may need to reheat the water, making sure that on these follow-up applications there is enough salt added to again have a saturated solution.

In many cases a peanut oil massage (sometimes referred to as a "rub") followed the Epsom salts pack. The area where the pack was placed was given special attention with the pure peanut oil during the massage.

DIRECTIONS FROM THE READINGS

For a twelve-year-old girl suffering from Wilms' tumor and a sarcoma growth on her left kidney (reading given on September 7, 1934):

> ... apply a pack of Epsom Salts—saturated solution. Let's have more of the heat than of the water; that is, the crash towel used for this pack would be saturated in the hot Epsom Salts solution but then wrung out—but have the solution in same so as to make for the superficial application of heat to the area, that would drive the Epsom Salts—so applied to the external system—into the active organisms of the system itself.   632-3

For a sixty-four-year-old woman with arthritis (reading given on October 20, 1941):

> In the present we would use the Epsom Salts Packs; either these or the Epsom Salts Baths. For the body in the present we would use first the Epsom Salts Packs, over the hands, elbows, knees and feet particularly; saturated solution of Epsom Salts; using heavy, large towels wrung out

of a saturated solution of Epsom Salts as hot as the body can stand
same. Wrap up the areas in them, you see; changing them about every
half hour for two to three hours each day.

After such Packs are used, massage the areas thoroughly with Peanut Oil—all that the body will absorb. Do this each time after a series
of the Packs. If the Packs are used more than once a day, then use the
Peanut Oil more than once also.   1512-3

For an adult male with spinal subluxations, neuritis, some paralysis
on the right side of his body, nephritis, and pain in neck and shoulder
areas (reading given on February 25, 1932):

> . . . The relaxing of the cerebro-spinal, especially from the 9th dorsal to
> the base of the brain, with a saturated solution of Epsom Salts (in
> packs), applied along the spine *before* the manipulations are given,
> will ease the body materially—and allow the manipulations to be more
> effective for the muscular forces, for the removal of the pressures in
> the segments along the upper dorsal and cervical area. These need not
> be applied unless there is the tautness . . .   4175-1

TESTIMONIALS/RESULTS

Similar to several other recommended remedies, the follow-up reports mention only that the reading was followed, but no specific mention is made of the particular remedy. Here are a few reports, though,
that noted the Epsom salts packs:

A fifty-five-year-old woman with rheumatoid tendencies, anemia,
general debilitation, and incoordination of eliminations wrote to Cayce
eight days after her reading:

> "Today I take up my pen again to tell you that I have taken up the
> threads of life once more . . . {*The pill doctor's*} capsules set my stom-
> ach afire . . . So, when we got your reading, the Epsom Salts packs
> helped immediately. Dr. Kraus [Eugene R. Kraus, D.O.] was very much
> worried, but he helped me on my feet again. We had quite an argument
> over you, but he said he saw things differently and was willing to follow

your reading, so all went well . . . "   325-17, Report #1

The woman had asked in her reading how the Epsom salts packs should be given, and the answer stated that whenever there was a " . . . return of the burning or heaviness in the stomach and in the chest . . . " the packs should be applied. (325-17)

The mother of a fifteen-year-old girl who received several readings from Cayce and who had suffered an appendicitis attack noted in a September 17, 1931, letter regarding her daughter:

" . . . The Epsom Salts Packs relieved some of the soreness . . . "
259-6, Report #2

One forty-six-year-old woman governess with multiple sclerosis did not have any success with the packs. Three months after her third reading she wrote on September 25, 1939:

" . . . I discontinued the Epsom Salts Packs, feeling worse after them. The sciatic nerve in my left leg began to be very painful. This added to my crampy feeling, difficulty to stretch it and great stiffness. I have also much trouble in keeping my balance, especially if I want to turn.
"Otherwise I am well and look fine and happy . . . "
1865-3, Report #3

Nearly two weeks later she had her fourth and final reading on October 6, 1939. Two months later she wrote:

"Since the end of October, I began to have new and more severe pain in my legs, though I followed faithfully your suggestions. {*She was introduced to Christian Science by a friend of hers and*} found much logic and help in it . . . it came clearly in my mind, that I was on the right way and feel I have to tell it to you, thanking you for what you did for me."
1865-4, Report #3

Cayce responded to her letter:

" . . . I am happy to know that you have that as answers to your needs.
There is *power* in *His* name, as in no other and may His blessings keep
you and give you just that as is needed to fill every atom of your being
with *love* and *hope*. Know I will be glad to hear from you at any and all
times, and can we ever be of a help, know we are glad to do so . . . "

1865-4, Report #4

ADDITIONAL INFORMATION

Epsom salts are a white, crystallized salt, used as a cathartic and as a
soaking aid for minor ailments. Epsom salts may also be taken orally as
a laxative. In the mid–eighteenth century the salts were widely used as
a purgative to help reduce swelling.

Chemically, Epsom salt is hydrated magnesium sulfate ($MgSO_4 \cdot 7H_2O$).
A member of the salt family, it gets its name from a city in southern
England, Epsom, where the salts were originally obtained from the
water of a mineral spring there. It is a one–hundred–percent natural
mineral.

OTHER USES FOR EPSOM SALTS

In the Cayce readings, the term Epsom salts is mentioned over eight
hundred times for a variety of uses: as a pack, for a fume bath, in a tub
or sitz bath, or to be taken internally as a laxative. For further information on these uses, see the chapters on "Epsom Salts Bath," "Steam/Fume
Bath," and "Sitz Bath."

Exercise

Most of us understand and agree with the importance of exercise, yet it takes additional effort and willingness to actually apply the knowledge, putting it into practice. Cayce gave many readings on this topic, encompassing the physical structure of the body from head to toe. One of the most well known in this family of health practices is the head and neck exercise, recommended to nearly three hundred individuals with a range of health concerns. The readings also offer a variety of perspectives on the importance of breathing, noting in several instances how poorly we perform this life–giving task. What follows is a fuller explanation of the use of these two exercises.

HEAD AND NECK EXERCISE

INDICATIONS

Brain lesion, bronchitis, cataracts, catarrh, detoxification, ear problems, eye problems, glandular disturbances, headaches, head noises, hearing difficulties, mastoiditis, myopia, nervousness, nervous system incoordination, osteochondritis, pelvic disorders, poor circulation, poor eliminations, sinusitis, speaking difficulties, spinal subluxations, stress, tendency toward deafness, tinnitus, tonsillitis, varicose veins, vertigo

MATERIALS NEEDED
Stool or chair—to sit upon when doing the exercise (you may also stand)

FREQUENCY OF APPLICATION
Regularly; each morning and evening
Move head 3 to 5 times in each direction

WHEN TO DO THE EXERCISE
Mornings (standing position) and evenings (sitting position), when walking out in the open, as a preparation for meditation

LENGTH OF TIME OF APPLICATION
One to 3 minutes; 2 to 3 weeks, then once a week for 2 to 3 weeks, then once a month, then repeat; 6 months

EXPECTED EFFECTS/PURPOSES
Improves nerve functioning and circulation in the head and neck
Relieves muscle tension and " . . . the pressures of the toxic forces . . . ". (3549-1)
Stimulates the thyroid
Improves circulation to the entire face, head, mouth, teeth, and neck
Keeps the throat and jaw line firm
Prevents the formation of double or multiple chins

DIRECTIONS
The movements of the head and neck exercise vary slightly from one reading to another. Some readings direct the individual to do the exercise, as if the technique were already well known. Newcomers to A.R.E. are usually introduced to the exercise in the Search for God Study Group, where it is taught as a preparation for meditation, though it was not specifically mentioned in the readings for that purpose. (See *Additional Information*.)

Usually one sits when doing the exercise, since, at least in the beginning, one may feel dizzy if one is standing up. The spine should be fairly straight. All movements are done slowly and effortlessly while one breathes mindfully throughout the exercise.

Bend the head forward, as if trying to touch your chin to your chest. Repeat three times. Then bend the head backward three times, extending it as far back as is comfortably possible. Next, bend to the right three times, as if you are trying to touch your ear to your shoulder. Then bend the head to the left three times. Now rotate the head fully around; begin by dropping the chin toward the chest, then make a circle, going first clockwise (to the right) three times, and then counterclockwise (to the left) three times.

Do this exercise morning and evening regularly, taking one to three minutes to finish. All the movements are done without force, taking one's time, and maintaining a comfort level throughout.

In the following readings' excerpts, you will note the slight variety in the steps of the exercise.

DIRECTIONS FROM THE READINGS

For a forty-two-year-old woman with spinal subluxations as well as ear and eye problems (reading given on April 20, 1932):

> Every morning and evening, for one to two minutes, take the head and neck exercise; that is, begin—sitting erect, either before arising or just after arising, and just before retiring or when ready to retire—with the head bend forward three times, just as far as it may be bent; slow, not fast. Then bend backward. Then to the left, then to the right—three times each one. Then circulate to the right three times, then circulate to the left three times. At first this will make some dizziness. It will, after a few days, make for a change in the hearing, producing at first rather inconvenience, but gradually will this be an aid to eyes, ears, nose, taste, and the general condition of the system.   413-2

For a thirty-four-year-old woman with myopia as well as neuritis (reading given on January 14, 1944):

(Q) How can I improve my vision?

(A) When we remove the pressures of the toxic forces we will improve the vision. Also the head and neck exercise will be most helpful. Take this regularly, not taking it sometimes and leaving off sometimes, but each morning and each evening take this exercise regularly for six months and we will see a great deal of difference: Sitting erect, bend the head forward three times, to the back three times, to the right side three times, to the left side three times, and then circle the head each way three times. Don't hurry through with it but take the time to do it. You will get results.   3549-1

For an adult male suffering with nasal catarrh (reading given on March 18, 1936):

Of morning upon arising take the head and neck exercise; circulating the head first, very slowly, three to five times to the right, then three to five times to the left. Sitting or standing erect, bend the head *backward* slowly, just as far as it can, three times; then forward three times; then to the left three times; then to the right three times. Take the *time* to do these, slowly but definitely; not as rote but as doing an act for the accomplishing of a purpose.   1131-3

For a forty-four-year-old man with a prolapsed Eustachian tube (reading given on June 5, 1938):

. . . we would take the head and neck exercise consistently; not just take it one day and forget it the next, or take it once a week or three to four times a week and leave off, but take it morning and evening—two to three minutes. This will add materially to the ability to keep the equal balance, and it will prevent much of those inclinations for the body to *feel* the heaviness through the upper portion of the system. That is: Sit very erect. Move the head forward two to three times, then a circular motion; then to the left or to the right; then to the rear, and then the circular motion again. Do this gently, positively. Not just to be gotten through with, but for *definite* activity to be received.   1564-2

TESTIMONIALS/RESULTS

A chiropractic doctor, Frank Moeser, sent in this report on October 17, 1949, in reference to reading 413-2 (see *Directions from the Readings*):

> "I have used this head and neck exercise for two cases of brachial neuralgia with one hundred percent results."   413-2, Report #10

Mrs. Vera Harrison of Virginia Beach, VA, wrote to the A.R.E. on November 14, 1966, commenting on her success with the head and neck exercise:

> "I had worn glasses for twenty-seven years. Last July an A.R.E. member saw me straining over the small print in a book on the table. She told me about the head and neck exercise in the Cayce readings and I started it immediately, once in the morning on a walk and once in the evening sitting very straight. Well, last week I threw my glasses away. The telephone book used to be dreaded like a plague and now I can read the smallest print in the Bible without glasses. I just thought other members ought to know about it."   3549-1, Report #8

Mrs. [5197], who was fifty-six years old when she received a Cayce reading on May 26, 1944, replied to a follow-up questionnaire in her letter of January 29, 1952:

> " . . . For a number of years prior to my reading, I had trouble all the time with my ear. It abscessed every few months. The last time, the doctor-specialist told me I would never hear more than 50% out of it. Several months later, I began the neck and head exercise. I went to this same specialist to have my glasses changed and asked him to look at my ear. He was amazed to see how normal it was, and said the 'hole' in the eardrum (which he told me would never close) was healed and closed. I told him of the head and neck exercise, but nothing more. 'No comment.' . . . Incidentally, I can hear my watch tick as clearly with my 'bad' ear as I can with the other one . . . "   5197-1, Report #3

ADDITIONAL INFORMATION

On January 16, 1976, Gladys Davis Turner, secretary of the A.R.E., wrote a letter to clarify some discussion regarding the head and neck exercise being used as a preparation for meditation. She commented:

" . . . As to the use of the head and neck exercises before meditation, this did not come in the meditation readings. I can remember no reference to this being a part of the meditation procedure other than the suggestion that we attune our bodies and prepare for meditation as indicated in the chapter on meditation—at the beginning of the book *A Search for God*. The head and neck exercises were given in physical readings for many people, myself included. It was supposed to stimulate the circulation and aid the whole sensory system, the eyes, the ears, etc. There were literally hundreds and hundreds of recommendations in the readings for use of the head and neck exercise . . .

"As I understand it, someone suggested at a conference many years ago that the entire group in the class take the head and neck exercise, during a break, just to loosen up or relax from sitting so long. This became a habit and it was recommended from the platform, or by the leader of the discussion or meditation period, so that it came to be done regularly as a part of the relaxing to prepare for meditation. This is very good I think, but I can't find a reading that definitely says that the head and neck exercise should be a part of the meditation procedure.

"The readings on meditation *do* say that the individual should do beforehand *whatever* will, for him, cleanse the body and the mind before entering meditation . . . "   470-37, Report #3

BREATHING EXERCISES

Actions that we perform automatically are those we frequently take for granted. Such is the case with the function of our respiratory system, which keeps us inhaling and exhaling without our having to focus on or think about it.

The readings mention how infrequently we breathe as deeply as we should, even suggesting to some individuals that they need to be trained in breathwork with accompanying exercises to practice taking deep breaths.

INDICATIONS

Asthma, cataracts, cough, dry throat, elephantiasis, fatigue, goiter, heaviness (across small of back), hypothyroidism, impaired speech, pelvic disorders, poor assimilations, poor circulation, scars on lungs, shortness of breath, sinusitis, streptococcus, tuberculosis

MATERIALS NEEDED

Stool or chair—to sit upon when doing the exercise (some are done standing or walking)

FREQUENCY OF APPLICATION

Daily; twice a day; 3 to 4 times during one session; 3 times, rest 5 minutes, then repeat; do sessions 3 times a week

WHEN TO DO THE EXERCISES

Mornings (before an open window) and evenings, during long walks morning and evening, " . . . in the *sunlight* as much as possible." (900-467), after series of spinal adjustments

LENGTH OF TIME OF APPLICATION

Three to 5 minutes, 5 to 6 minutes

EXPECTED EFFECTS/PURPOSES

Clarifies and purifies the system
Purifies the blood that circulates through the lungs
Enhances circulation
Increases oxygen production

DIRECTIONS

Although there are variations for this exercise, what is fairly consistent is that as one rises on the toes, lifting the hands above the head, one inhales, breathing in through the nostrils; when returning to a standing position, lowering the arms, one exhales, breathing out through the mouth. In one reading, though—288-40—the breathing sequence is reversed.

Some individuals were advised to stoop over or bend forward, toward the floor, after rising on the toes, being able eventually, with a little practice, to touch the floor with one's fingertips while remaining on the toes.

In some readings, exhalations through the mouth were to be done suddenly, to help expel the carbon dioxide from the lungs and fill them with fresh air, " . . . unless—of course—one is breathing dust or pollen or some disturbing factor; but this is presupposing that the body is breathing fresh air, see?" . . . (1158-31)

Any further instructions can be noted in the *Directions from the Readings* section.

DIRECTIONS FROM THE READINGS

For a thirty-seven-year-old male with lumbago and tendencies toward neuritis and rheumatism (reading given on May 26, 1942):

(Q) Outline breathing exercises best for purifying the body.
(A) Three to five minutes of morning and evening—before an open window, of course—that of rising on the toes with the hands gradually raised above the head at the same time, breathing in deeply. The better way is to breathe first through one nostril, then the other, but this is not easily done—in the beginning. This is the best exercise that may be taken by most any body. For this is not only an exercise of the respiratory system but of all the muscular forces. Watch a cat or a tiger as it stretches. That is the exercise for the muscular forces.

If there is the attempt to vary the breathing from the right to the left nostril, keep same balanced. The left nostril is the spiritual, or the easing; the right nostril is the strength. So keep 'em balanced! Don't get too much strength—that is, don't get more physical strength than you are able to keep balanced through the system. Two to three times through each nostril is the better way, for the expansion of the lungs and for the purifying of circulation by same. Breathe *in* through the nostril, *out* through the mouth—when taking such exercise.   2533-3

For a twenty–nine–year–old woman with sinusitis and pelvic disorders (reading given on February 10, 1938):

> Of morning, and upon arising especially (and don't sleep too late!)—
> and before dressing, so that the clothing is loose or the fewer the bet-
> ter—standing erect before an open window, breathe deeply; gradually
> raising hands *above* the head, and then with the circular motion of the
> body from the hips bend forward; breathing *in* (and through the nos-
> trils) as the body rises on the toes—breathing very deep; *exhaling sud-
> denly* through the *mouth; not* through the nasal passages. Take these
> for five to six minutes. Then as these progress, gradually *close* one of
> the nostrils (even if it's necessary to use the hand—but if it is closed
> with the left hand, raise the right hand; and when closing the right
> nostril with the right hand, then raise the left hand) *as* the breathing
> *in* is accomplished. Rise, and the circular motion of the body from the
> hips, and bending forward; *expelling* as the body reaches the lowest
> level in the bending towards the floor (expelling through the mouth,
> suddenly). See?   1523-2

For a twenty–seven–year–old woman suffering from nervous system incoordination (reading given on July 3, 1933):

> (Q) What breathing exercises would be best for me?
> (A) Those that *should* be the activity to every well-balanced body. Morn-
> ing and evening exercises with the full and deep inhalation, and quick
> exhalation from the lungs; breathing in through the nostrils and ex-
> haling through the mouth quickly.   369-10

TESTIMONIALS/RESULTS

No material exists in the Reports section of the readings on "breathing exercise(s)." Certainly members of Search for God Study Groups continue to use this exercise along with the head and neck exercise prior to
meditation. Perhaps the lack of information reflects this quote from the
readings:

. . . few ever consider the necessity of breathing or the lack of same to keep alive. These are just as much a portion of body, mind, soul . . .

                                                    3125-2

An additional comment to be made here: Besides the exercises described in the few selections in this chapter, there remain other breathing exercises given for individuals to perform. The index to the readings lists over fifty references, only a few of which are included here.

ADDITIONAL INFORMATION

The following is an excerpt from the Prayer Group series of readings (the 281 series), given for the Glad Helpers and describing the breathing exercise:

> Then, as one formula—not the only one, to be sure—for an individual that would enter into meditation for self, for others:
> Cleanse the body with pure water. Sit or lie in an easy position, without binding garments about the body. Breathe in through the right nostril three times, and exhale through the mouth. *Breathe* in three times through the left nostril and exhale through the right. Then, either with the aid of a low music, or the incantation of that which carries self deeper—deeper—to the seeing, feeling, experiencing of that image in the creative forces of love, enter into the Holy of Holies . . .
>
>   281-13

These breathing exercises take very little time to perform—a few minutes during the morning and evening hours, and keep us in better balance while rejuvenating our bodies through increased circulation and better eliminations.

> Let each individual know that it came into life with a purpose from God. Let each individual know that it is as a harp upon which the breath of God would play.   281-60

Glyco-Thymoline Pack

If there is any one remedy that is a "must" for the proverbial medicine cabinet, a bottle of Glyco–Thymoline would rank near the top of the list. Some people may be unfamiliar with this product, which was first manufactured in 1878 and was readily available during the time Edgar Cayce was giving readings—and is still obtainable today. Probably because of its availability as well as its beneficial formula, it was often suggested by the sleeping Cayce for a variety of applications. The word *Glyco* occurs over 1,200 times in the text of the readings: to be used as an intestinal antiseptic, orally or during colonics; for nasal or throat sprays; as a gargle; in ear or eye syringes; and in douches. The manufacturer also recommends its use for oral hygiene (mouthwash, gargle, cleaning dentures), personal hygiene (cleansing external anal and genital areas), and for certain skin conditions (poison ivy, stings, bites, burns, chapped skin, sunburn). It is recommended in the readings for use both externally as a pack (with or without heat) and internally as an alkalizer and antiseptic for the body; depending upon how it is applied, it can be used either diluted or full strength.

A cautionary note is mentioned in *An Edgar Cayce Home Medicine*

Guide (p. 59): "When taking Glyco-Thymoline internally, it should be kept in mind that it is poisonous when taken in large quantities, and no more than a few drops daily should be taken." When using it as a mouthwash or gargle, those concerned about the accidental swallowing of it need not worry. " . . . gargling each evening and morning with Glyco-Thymoline . . . will aid, and if a little of it is swallowed it will not hurt." (1688-9)

INDICATIONS

(External application) Bites, bladder ailments, burns, catarrh, chapped skin, common cold, congestion, denture cleaning, eye problems (irritated, tired), goiter, personal hygiene, poison ivy, poor digestion, postnasal drip, prior to adjustments, sinusitis, stings, sunburn

(Internal application) Acidity, bad breath, ear problems, intestinal disturbances, mucosity, nasal and throat catarrh, oral hygiene, throat irritations

CONTRAINDICATIONS

Check the ingredients (see *Additional Information*) for the possibility of allergic reactions to any of these items listed; caution—use internally as an alkalizer only under the supervision of your health care professional, avoiding excessive amounts, " . . . for an overalkalinity is much more harmful than a little tendency occasionally for acidity . . . " (808-3)

MATERIALS NEEDED

Glyco-Thymoline—16-fluid-ounce bottle (473 ml)

Gauze, cotton cloth, towel, or washcloth—for compresses in external applications; also used to cleanse area following the pack

Throat sprayer—for use with throat irritations

Fountain syringe—for use in vaginal douches; 2 tablespoons Glyco-Thymoline per 1 quart of water

Eyecup—for use in eye irritations or problems; 2 parts water (preferably distilled) to 1 part Glyco-Thymoline

Warm water—to bathe off area after removal of pack

Small cup, bowl, or container—to hold warm water for cleaning area after pack

Electric heating pad, hot water bottle, or salt pack (optional)—to maintain heat

Oil cloth, plastic, or towel (optional)—to place over the pack as a compress, or under the area or limb where the pack is applied in order to protect the sheets

FREQUENCY OF APPLICATION
Daily, 2 to 3 times daily, 3 to 4 times a week

AMOUNT OF DOSAGE
In small amount of water: 2 to 15 drops; full strength: for mouthwash and gargle; in compresses

LENGTH OF TIME OF APPLICATION
(External applications) 5 to 10 minutes; 15 to 20 minutes; 20 to 30 minutes to 1 hour; 1½ to 2 hours; 3 to 4 evenings in succession; 10 days, off 5 days, then repeat; " . . . until the {nasal or sinus} passages are clear . . . " (2794-2); take internally for a " . . . sufficient period until the *odor* of same may be detected from the stool . . . " (1807-3); " . . . until the system has been purified . . . " (2794-2)

LOCATION OF APPLICATION
Abdomen, across sacral area, across the face, across the hips, base and side of the ear, knee, over affected area, over lumbar and sacral areas, over nasal passages, over the eyes, spinal column (before adjustments), throat

SIZE OF PACK
Large enough to cover affected area, 2 to 5 thicknesses

WHEN TO APPLY THE PACK
Evenings, the day before spinal adjustments, " . . . whenever there is any distress . . . " (2794-2)

EXPECTED EFFECTS/PURPOSES

Alkalizes and purifies the alimentary canal
Treats mucosity
Acts as an intestinal antiseptic
Purifies reproductive organs
Breaks up formation of cataracts
Aids in elimination (kidneys, bladder, pelvic organs)
Assists the system to absorb poisons
Relaxes spine the day before adjustments
Reduces inflammation
Relieves local tension

DIRECTIONS

To help the recipient of the reading prepare a Glyco–Thymoline pack, these general suggestions were sometimes included along with a copy of the individual's reading:

> " . . . Use 2 to 3 thicknesses of cotton cloth well saturated with the commercial strength Glyco-Thymoline and apply over affected areas, or areas specified for your particular case. An electric pad may be used to keep the Pack warm. A piece of oil cloth (or plastic) may be put over the Pack, after it is placed on body, to prevent soiling linens, etc. Apply for 20 to 30 minutes, to an hour at the time. In cold weather, place the bottle of Glyco-Thymoline in a pan of hot water to take the chill off before using it for the Pack."   2794-2, Report #4

The readings recommend using the packs for a wide variety of cases. In some instances an unheated pack is suggested, while in others heat is to be applied over the pack.

To use as a pack for sinusitis, for example, saturate a cotton cloth, gauze, or washcloth with full–strength Glyco–Thymoline. Warm the cloth with the Glyco by folding it onto a heating pad after covering it with a plastic sheet to protect the pad. One's face should be cleansed and free from makeup prior to the application. Lie down on a bed or lean back in a recliner and place the pack directly on the closed eyelids, covering as well the sides of the nose, the forehead, eyebrows, and cheekbones; in other words, cover the whole sinus cavity area of the face. On top of the pack place a piece of plastic or oil cloth, which slows the rate of evaporation. Heat can be maintained with a heating pad, a hot water bottle, an infrared lamp, or a salt pack. Leave the pack in place for 20 to 30 minutes. It may be reused a few times (keep it in a sealed plastic bag), and is then discarded.

Take a cotton cloth, gauze, or cotton balls and dip or soak them in warm water. Wipe the eye sockets, cheeks, and forehead gently to remove any residue or stickiness from the pack.

Repeat the pack application, if needed, until all traces of the condition are no longer present, up to two to three times a day.

An increase in discharge from the nose and throat passages is likely, since the Glyco causes the infected lining of the sinus cavities to cleanse themselves. To avoid further difficulties in the intestinal tract from these waste products, add a few drops of Glyco to your drinking water throughout the day.

DIRECTIONS FROM THE READINGS

For a fifty-year-old man with a goiter on his thyroid (reading given on February 19, 1943):

> Each evening we would apply locally, about the throat and neck, a pack of Glyco-Thymoline; that is, about three thicknesses of cloth—preferably old cotton cloth, that would reach around the whole of the neck, moistened with Glyco-Thymoline and applied warm; not warming the Glyco-Thymoline but warming the cloth after being moistened with the Glyco, see? Let this remain around the neck through the greater part of the evening, then bathe off the area with plain warm water. And the next evening apply the same. Do this for at least ten days. Then leave off a period of five days, and then do this again.   2864-2

For a thirty-four-year-old woman with sinusitis (reading given on May 19, 1943):

We would use the Glyco-Thymoline packs over the nasal passages, or sinus passages. Saturate three to four thicknesses of cotton cloth, or gauze, in warm Glyco-Thymoline, and apply over the passages, allowing such a pack to remain on for fifteen to twenty minutes at the time—and keep up until the passages are clear. Apply such packs whenever there is any distress—either in the sinus or in the digestive system. Such packs may also be applied over the abdominal area to advantage, as well as over the face, see?   2794-2

For a thirty–six–year–old woman whose system was too acidic (reading given on June 8, 1939):

Also we would use an alkalizer for the alimentary canal. Preferably . . . each day take three or four drops of Glyco-Thymoline internally, in a little water. Take this for sufficient period until the *odor* of same may be detected from the stool. This will purify the whole of the alimentary canal and create an alkaline reaction *through* the lower portion of the alimentary canal.   1807-3

TESTIMONIALS/RESULTS

Overall, the response has been positive. From Samuel E. Benesch in Baltimore, Maryland, comes this report collected as part of a compilation in July 1949:

"In 10 to 15 minutes I obtain relief from using the Glyco-Thymoline Packs for sinusitis. The pain is relieved completely, the sinus drains, and elimination shows definite improvement. I use the Packs directly over sinus (and abdomen when condition is acute). I use the Infra-Red bulb as a source of heat. This treatment alone pays for my A.R.E. membership in doctors' bills saved. The eyes are rested and strengthened. Since breath control is important in meditation, this system is extremely valuable to me in relieving bad sinus conditions . . . "
                    2794-2, Report #6

Another sinus condition account from the previous same compiled report was written by Mrs. [808], who received twenty readings from Cayce, from February 2, 1935, to May 3, 1944, when she was between twenty-seven and thirty-six years of age:

" . . . In February 1948 I received extracts from 2794-2 regarding Glyco-Thymoline Packs, when I was suffering with an awful attack, the fourth time that winter . . . It was rather messy, but—believe it or not—it opened the congestion in my sinuses and it was the first time I felt any relief. I continued for about a week and it cleared up completely.

"This past winter, whenever I'd feel an attack coming on I'd heat the Glyco-Thymoline in a glass custard dish set in boiling water and use the Packs as hot as I could stand over the temple. Then I put a piece of oil cloth over that, and the heating pad on top of that. I used this for ¾ of an hour. It would clear up immediately any persistent pain in that area and would require several days' treatment to clear up a severe sinus infection . . . "   2794-2, Report #6

In his waking state Cayce also encouraged others to try this remedy. In a letter on May 20, 1943, to Miss [2487] he remarked:

" . . . Haven't you gotten rid of that cold as yet—use Glyco packs over your face and neck, will take it right out . . . "   2487-2, Report #8

ADDITIONAL INFORMATION

A registered, trademarked name, Glyco-Thymoline contains natural ingredients and is manufactured by Kress and Owen Company, Inc., in Avondale Estates, Georgia. Its previous label stated: "Treatment for Mucosity," but its present label denotes it to be used for "Mouthwash and Oral Hygiene." Packaged in a 16-fluid-ounce bottle (473 ml), it lasts quite a while, even when taken on a regular basis, since most often it is used in small amounts or in diluted form. However, occasionally for oral hygiene and often for packs, for example, it may be used full strength. The manufacturer reports that, although the label was redesigned to conform to US Food and Drug Administration regulations, the formula has not changed since Cayce's time. Many directives for its use as given in the Cayce readings closely coincide with the manufacturer's recommendations.

What makes this formula so effective in relieving sinusitis? Eucalyptol, menthol, pine oil, thymol, and methyl salicylate (wintergreen) are some of the ingredients listed on the label. These are commonly used in preparations for liniments and vaporizers. There is also its distinctive red color, unfortunately mistaken for FD&C Red Dye #40 (or Red #40). Yet the source of this color, carmine (also called carminic acid), is a pigment with an unusual origin.

As a coloring agent used to provide a deep red shade to candies, shampoos, fruit juices, gelatins and other foodstuffs, beverages, and cosmetics, carmine and its close relative cochineal come from a particular South and Central American beetle known as *Dactylopius coccus*. Indigenous people in the Americas collected the female insects, immersed them in hot water to kill them and dissolve their waxy coatings, then dried them in the sun and ground them into a fine powder. The Spanish explorers recognized and admired the brilliant scarlet color with its extraordinary colorfast properties and began exporting the dried insects to Europe. About 70,000 insects make one pound of cochineal.

Because some synthetic dyes have proven dangerous to humans either when taken internally or when they seep into the skin through external applications, cochineal is widely used. Aside from a few cases of allergic reactions, it is a safe food colorant; however, because of Jewish dietary laws, it is not found in kosher products. Red #40, though bug-free, is actually derived from coal. Despite Western society's squeamishness that some of our favorite foods might contain beetle extract, it apparently causes no harm and is reportedly a safe coloring agent.

OTHER USES FOR GLYCO-THYMOLINE

For relieving *sinusitis,* in addition to applying a pack across the face, you may put it over the abdominal area at a different time. The pack may be applied whenever there is any distress—whether in the sinus cavities or in the digestive system. About twice a day, take Glyco-

Thymoline internally, placing two to four drops in half a glass of water. Keep this schedule up " . . . until the system has been purified . . . " (2794-2); that is, when the odor of Glyco is detected in the stool, in which case the body has had enough.

To restore the normal *acid-alkaline balance* in one's system, diluted Glyco-Thymoline was sometimes recommended: from two to fifteen drops in a small amount of water once a day. The dosage apparently varied with the degree of overacidity to be corrected and was taken upon arising in the morning, on an empty stomach, or during the day. When the system is overly acidic, according to the readings, cold and congestion can easily develop. Note also the caution to overalkalinity in the *Contraindications* section.

For *eye problems*, such as tired or irritated eyes, use an eye cup filled with two parts of (preferably) distilled water to one part of Glyco. The eye can be bathed in this weak solution when the filled cup is placed over the eye.

To cleanse the *secretions from the eyes* after an application of a potato poultice, bathe them with a soft cotton cloth or cotton balls soaked in half Glyco, half distilled water. This antiseptic will help remove any residue that is drawn from the eyes by the poultice. (*See also* the chapter "Potato Poultice.")

For a *sore throat*, to soothe and cleanse the irritated membranes, the manufacturer recommends gargling with Glyco or using a throat spray: two parts water to one part Glyco. The readings also recommend using a throat spray, but with full–strength, warm Glyco, twice a day—morning and evening. In several cases, alternating a throat with a nasal spray was suggested to alkalize and cleanse the system. One reading describes more detail about this combination:

> As a spray for the nasal passages and for the throat, use these alternately. For their effects are different yet their combining with the effects of the mucous membranes and the circulatory forces should keep and should create an elimination and a throwing off of these conditions . . .   1131-4

To help eliminate further excess poisons, the individual was to take the laxative Castoria followed by three to six drops of Glyco twice a day in half a glass of water. The spray, full strength, was to be taken in the evening, before retiring.

> . . . But do not use it as cold as the ordinary temperature, but have it about the temperature of the body. Put it in the bottle from which the spray is used (or atomizer) and place in warm water until it has about the temperature of the body. Spray this in the nasal passages (holding the head way back). Spray the throat with same.   1131-4

For use in an *ear syringe* for catarrh, Glyco-Thymoline was recommended in one reading, mixing half Glyco and half distilled water. " . . . This should be used warm—not hot, not cold—when used in an ear syringe or in a nasal atomizer." (2899-2)

A *nasal spray* for a fifty-four-year-old woman with "a chronic sinus disturbance" (1770-8) was suggested along with Glyco-Thymoline packs across her face. The spray was to be used twice a day with full-strength Glyco-Thymoline, and the packs applied two or three times a day with warm, full-strength Glyco, with two thicknesses. The reading clarified the temperature of the packs as well as offered some interesting comments:

> . . . we do not mean to use the *Glyco-Thymoline* hot but just sufficiently warm so that the heat causes the certain oils in the elements to loosen themselves, so as to enter into the cavities of the nasal passages and into those areas so distressed at times. For these are the source of those disturbances that cause quick pulsation of heart, or the slipping or skipping of the heart beat also.   1770-8

For *mucosity* one may use Glyco-Thymoline as often as needed to reduce the mucus—by gargling or spraying or rinsing the mouth—with the Glyco either diluted or used full strength. The readings also suggest taking Glyco internally two or three times a day: three to five drops in a glass of water, as an intestinal antiseptic.

If you are receiving a *colonic* (an irrigation or cleansing of the colon) as part of your therapy regimen, you may be able to request the addition of diluted Glyco–Thymoline in the final waters of your treatment. (In some states in the US additives to the water for colonics are prohibited.) The solution is made ahead of time (1 tablespoon Glyco to 1 or 1½ quarts of water; or 2 tablespoons Glyco to 1½ quarts of water) and introduced into the colon by means of a syringe. The Glyco helps release mucus from the system and acts as an intestinal antiseptic to purify the system and alkalize the body.

For *vaginal douches*, especially after one's menstrual period, Glyco–Thymoline is used as an antiseptic and purifier of the reproductive organs. The readings recommend a fountain syringe for the application, with one or two quarts of body–temperature water, adding two tablespoons of Glyco to each quart of water. In one case for hemorrhaging (2175–4), the douches were to be given at least twice a week.

As a remedy for *sunburn* (also recommended by its manufacturer), Glyco is mentioned in one reading along with several other items:

> . . . Any good lotion would be well for the sunburn; such as soda water {*water with a little baking soda added to it*}, or any application that would act as a balm, in the forms of some characters of oils that remove the fire from the affected areas—such as Glyco-Thymoline.
>
> 3051-1

(*See also* the chapter "Apple Cider Vinegar (and Salt) Pack" for information on applying vinegar to a sunburned skin.)

Several applications for getting rid of *dandruff* are given in this reading:

> Any of those preparations that are a good scalp cleansing tone; as Lavoris or Glyco-Thymoline—or combining these occasionally; and Fitch's Hair Restorer—which dissolves same, and is acid of course; while the first two named are alkaline—and these are well to be considered—the acid *and* alkaline reaction on the scalp. Of course, oil with Vaseline; that is, as an Olive Oil Shampoo, with Vaseline rubbed in afterwards is very well.   1523-3

In conclusion, Glyco-Thymoline is an effective remedy for a number of conditions. As an alkalizing agent, it provides a welcoming comfort and relief to bring one's body into better balance.

Grape Juice

Many juices that are derived from specific vegetables, fruits, and meats are mentioned in the readings for their value as a form of medicine or tonic, concurring with the popular idea that food has a medicinal benefit in one's healing process. Onions, potato peelings, liver, beef, and grapes are all mentioned as sources of these juices, to be consumed along with and in conjunction with other modalities.

To control weight increase, over one hundred readings suggest " . . . the grape juice way, rather than any particular dieting; {and} just requiring that the body refrain from too much sweets and starches." (470-32) Instead of following a strict diet, leaving out specific foods, the readings emphasize a more balanced approach with reductions and some elimination of food groups as part of one's dietary regimen. To reduce weight gain and help control one's appetite, individuals were advised to drink diluted grape juice—taken three or four times a day—thirty minutes before each meal and again at bedtime. How much juice in proportion to water varies only slightly from one reading to another. For individuals struggling with this imbalance, the incentive and potentially successful results may be worth the effort.

INDICATIONS

Appetite control, better eliminations, intestinal disorders, intestinal gas, obesity, peritonitis, strengthener for the body, toxemia

MATERIALS NEEDED

Fresh grapes (to press out the juice)—Concord grapes preferred or fresh Welch's Grape Juice; unsweetened; " . . . not those fermented or those that have been canned . . . " (1045-8)

Plain water—to dilute the juice; only one reading recommended carbonated water (470-21); another reading recommended ginger ale or half-carbonated and half plain water (942-1)

Instrument for mashing the grapes

Strainer—to separate juice from pulp and seeds

Container—in which to place fresh juice

FREQUENCY OF DOSAGE

Once or twice daily, 3 or 4 times a day—30 minutes before each meal and at bedtime (most frequent recommendation), sipped slowly

AMOUNT OF DOSAGE

Sips; small amounts; small glass; 2 or 3 teaspoons; 1 ounce daily; 1 to 2 ounces during day; *ratio of grape juice to water:* 2 to 3 ounces of grape juice: 1 ounce of plain water; ¾ of a glass of juice: ¼ of a glass of water; ⅔ juice: ⅓ water; 1½ ounces juice: ½ ounce water; 1 ounce juice: 1½ ounces water; 1½ to 2 ounces juice: a little water; 3 ounces juice: 1 ounce water; equal amounts: 4 ounces juice: 4 ounces water; 4 ounces juice: 6 ounces water; " . . . later, there may be mixed orange juice with same, half and half . . . " (852- 6)

LENGTH OF TIME OF APPLICATION

At least 1 month or 6 weeks, leave off 2 to 3 weeks, then take another 6-week period; about 4 weeks, leave off 2 weeks, then repeat; several weeks, off 1 or 2 weeks, then repeat; 5 to 10 days

EXPECTED EFFECTS/PURPOSES

Reduces weight and excess sugar

Helps with eliminations

Prevents desire for excessive starches and sweets

Helps to maintain normal balance in weight

Supplies beneficial sugar to the system (without weight gain)

Assists in controlling the appetite

Reduces the desire for foods that cause weight gain

Gives " . . . strength to the vitality of the resistance forces in the body."

(1183-2)

DIRECTIONS

Mash and crush the fresh grapes, squeezing enough juice from them for the amount you wish to drink. Strain the mixture, collecting only the juice—no seeds or pulp.

Amounts of juice range from small sips to three-fourths of a glass (see *Amount of Dosage*) and should be made just prior to drinking it, according to the readings. The grapes to be used are the same as those for the poultice—preferably the Concord grapes (*see also* the chapter on "Grape Poultice" for further information). However, " . . . If the juice from fresh grapes is found to be impractical, then take the fresh Welch's Grape Juice." (1224-3)

Whether using fresh grapes or Welch's, the juice is usually slightly diluted with plain water; only one reading recommended carbonated water for the mixture. (For differences in the ratio of juice to water, see *Amount of Dosage*.) The slightly diluted juice is to be sipped slowly, not gulped down. " . . . Take about five to ten minutes to drink the juice each time . . . ," one reading (1431-2) suggested.

For the majority of cases the recommended period for drinking the juice is thirty minutes before each meal and again before retiring in the evening—so four times total. Once or twice daily is suggested a few times for different individuals. " . . . Even though the meal may consist only of a glass of orange juice and a piece of toast, or the like, take the grape juice thirty minutes beforehand—and at bedtime . . . " (257-217)

For how long to carry out this regimen, see *Length of Time of Application.*

DIRECTIONS FROM THE READINGS

For an eighteen-year-old girl suffering from peritonitis (reading given on September 23, 1935):

> *Then* there may be a little stimulation given in the crushed grapes; that is, the juice only of crushed grapes. Not the same as used for the poultice {*recommended as a treatment for her as well*}, but the same character of grapes as used for the poultice. The colder this may be the better . . .
>
> . . . begin with the grape juice (from the crushed fresh grapes, not grape juice that has been allowed to stand). This may be strained; not seasoned with sugar or the like, but just the natural fresh juice. Gradually, later, there may be mixed orange juice with same, half and half, but use the grape juice first—from the fresh crushed grapes . . .
>
> 852-6

For a twenty-five-year-old woman with scleroderma and a weight problem (reading given on May 19, 1944):

> That there has been a general or great increase in the weight of the body is not too well, but if we would begin with these by the month, we may reduce the weight without injury to the recuperating forces being set up in the body. Do begin and take for a month, and leave it off for some several weeks and again try, ½ hour before each meal and before retiring, 3 oz. of grape juice with 1 oz. of plain water; and do not eat sweets, but more of fresh vegetables cooked and raw, and not too much of any kind of bread, though whole grain cereals may be taken and used as a supplement for bread.   2514-15

For a seventy-four-year-old woman suffering from obesity and toxemia (reading given on April 20, 1940):

> (Q) Is it important to reduce weight? How much and by what means?
> (A) It is more important that an equal *balance* be kept. As we find, the weight may be reduced some *without* disturbance; and as we find, the

better manner would be through the refraining from breads or greases of any kind, of course, and by the taking of Grape Juice—preferably the juice from fresh grapes, this prepared at the time to be taken, three times each day; taking about an ounce and a half to two ounces (diluted with a little water) half an hour before each meal. If the juice from fresh grapes is found to be impractical, then take the fresh Welch's Grape Juice.   1224-3

TESTIMONIALS/RESULTS

A twenty-five-year-old optometrist, Mrs. [259], wrote on October 6, 1942:

"Welch's Grape Juice has triumphed again! The reading in January put me on it and since then I've lost fifteen pounds. It was gradual enough so that it was hardly noticeable but when I stepped on the scales at Dr. Sellers' yesterday we just couldn't believe it. The doctor made me get off and he checked the scales for balance to be sure it was right . . . "   259-10, Report #4

Two years before, she had written: "I'm getting too fat and must start taking exercise to reduce." (259-7, Report #16) Cayce teasingly wrote back: "You'd better try the Welch's Grape Juice way. It works if you are man enough to live up to it . . . " (Report #17)

In another letter that Cayce wrote on April 17, 1939, mention was made of successful outcomes others had with the grape juice. Mrs. [1829] was advised to try the diet:

" . . . for reducing. Take about two ounces of Welch {sic} grape juice and one ounce of water half {an} hour before the noon and evening meal and at bedtime. Believe in a few weeks you will see a lot of difference. Some to whom this has been given {have} lost as much as twenty pounds in three months, and {it} hasn't made them weak either. Yes, there was a lady here yesterday afternoon, said she had lost forty pounds in last four months and just feels fine, looks lots better also.

> "Do hope you will soon be feeling a whole lot better—try grape
> juice. Think you will like it . . . "   1829-2, Report #2

A thirty-five-year-old musician received a health reading on December 14, 1940. He was advised to take the grape juice diet for his weight problem, among other recommendations. Following his reading's suggestions, he continued to lose weight. Two years later in a follow-up questionnaire, in answer to the question, "Describe the extent to which improvements have resulted," he wrote, "Lost about 130 lbs. most of which was fat . . . " (2421-1 Report #6)

ADDITIONAL INFORMATION
Over forty readings mention Welch's Grape Juice by name, ten of which refer to it as "preferable" to other brands or to be used if freshly crushed grapes are unavailable. A notation made at the end of reading 457-7 summarizes Cayce's idea of " . . . Welch's Grape Juice as the purest of the more well-known varieties on the market."

Why is it preferable? Here are several comments from the readings:

> . . . The Welch's . . . has more of the elements in same that aid in the
> reduction of the carbohydrates in the system—and thus tends to sup-
> ply the food values in a way that is in keeping with that which has been
> indicated as the purpose for taking same . . .   1309-3

The grape juice is also "unfermented" (459-11) and " . . . will make for better assimilation, better eliminations, and better conditions throughout the system." (2067-3)

It is also "Prepared without benzoate of soda {*a preservative*} . . . " (470-19)

The Web site for Welch's states that they have been in the grape business since 1869. The juice is "made from freshly ripened purple Concord grapes from Welch's own vineyards and contains no artificial additives, preservatives, or sweeteners. It is also fat free, cholesterol free, and naturally rich in antioxidants." (Antioxidants help support the heart and the body's immune system.) Each glassful contains two servings of fruit with 100 percent Daily Value of vitamin C.

The number one cause of being overweight is eating excess starch; and the sugars that come from these starches are addictive, even at the cellular level. Substituting a sugar that does not support the addiction will help offset this imbalance. One reading describes it this way:

> . . . if the grape juice is taken it supplies a sugar, the kind of sugar though that works with the system—that which is necessary, see? and then that prevents the system's desire for starches and sweets in excess. Not that these are not to be taken at all, for they supply, of course, the necessary heat units for the body in a great measure; but as these would be supplied through the taking of the grape juice, or the eating of the grapes (if they are taken *as* the regular diet, and not just occasionally), there would only be the partaking of others as the appetite calls for same. When the appetite is controlled, it will govern the necessary forces in these directions.   470-19

In addition to reducing the consumption of sweets and starches, drinking diluted grape juice " . . . will reduce the excess sugar. Though {there} is sugar in the grape juice, it is a different character and will produce a better reaction through the alimentary canal . . . " (1170-3) When the cravings are under better control, one can eat a more healthful diet.

Grape juice in and of itself, of course, cannot stand alone in reducing weight. Receiving osteopathic manipulations, colonics, and steam baths also help to " . . . keep down the weight as well as remove poisons." (3413-2) Exercise and good nutrition are also important adjuncts to reducing. " . . . if the Grape Juice is taken, we will find the diet will adjust itself . . . " (1812-1); " . . . the appetite will change a great deal." (1309-2), Cayce told another. The person will come to eat, then, what the body really calls for and needs.

OTHER USES FOR GRAPES

In addition to drinking diluted grape juice for weight control, fresh grapes play a prominent role in the Cayce healing regimen (mentioned over two hundred times in the text of the readings): as an abdominal poultice for a variety of bowel and intestinal disturbances (see the chapter "Grape Poultice") and as an adjunct to one's normal diet.

Recommended in over thirty readings is a type of mono-diet: eating only grapes—as many as you want—without the seeds for three or four days, preferably the purple variety or Concord grape. Sometimes the diet was done in conjunction with the grape poultice: " . . . And during those three to four days {of eating only grapes} we would apply the grape poultices across all of the abdomen itself." (683-3) In a few readings, milk was added to the grape diet: " . . . Milk of mornings and evenings . . . Milk and grapes for three days as the diet." (977-1)

The principal reason for following the grape diet was for its laxative effect. An adult woman with an impacted colon and suffering from indigestion was told:

> We would be most mindful that there are the diets that tend to keep towards the laxative nature, rather than an acid or tending to make for a tendency towards constipation. Hence we would have a great deal, or great quantities at times of citrus fruit juices—and at other periods quantities of grapes. Let there be days when the whole day's food value would be only grapes; not with the seed, but these well masticated. Having whole periods when there would be such activities to make for the cleansing and changing of the toxic forces (that make for those pressures in the activities of the whole system throughout) will overcome these tendencies.   747-1

Grapes, as well as citrus fruits and most vegetables, when taken internally, are alkaline-reacting in the body, helping combat the buildup of acidity which may cause colds, weaken our defense system, and make us more vulnerable to sickness and disease.

Grapes also contain potassium, phosphorus, calcium, iron, magnesium, and other minerals as well as vitamins A, B_1, B_2, B_6, C, and K. The readings describe them as "blood-building" foods.

An interesting comment from Cayce in his waking state, mentioned briefly in the chapter on "Grape Poultice," is his reply to a query from a seventy-three-year-old executive, who wrote on August 26, 1943:

> "It is my understanding that members may ask questions from time to time, and so receive answers through you from the other side. If I am right in this, I would like to ask the following ... Are grapes and the juice of grapes properly extracted one of the best healing foods, breaking down toxic growth, allowing *nature* to complete the healing of the physical body? ... "
>
> 1942-3, Report #4

Cayce replied:

> " ... while {*I*} cannot properly give you as complete an answer to your questions as you would like, without a lot of research in the files, will give you my personal opinion on same from what {*I*} have absorbed from the information presented on these subjects ... Fresh Grape Juice properly extracted is one of the best healing foods for any intestinal disorder, and does reduce intestinal toxic poisons ... "
>
> 1942-3, Report #5

It is interesting to have Cayce's opinion as gleaned from his years of perusing his own trance readings.

Grape Poultice

By definition, a poultice consists of any soft mass, such as mustard, herbs, flour, potatoes, or clay, that is spread or placed on a cloth, towel, or gauze and applied to the body; it can be warm, moist, hot, or cool.

Recommended in nearly forty readings, the grape poultice, like the more familiar castor oil pack, is also placed over the abdomen to relieve a variety of discomforts associated with various bowel diseases or disturbances. Instead of wool flannel—as in the castor oil pack—the grape poultice uses gauze, cheesecloth, or heavy cloth to contain the bulk of grapes and hold them on the abdomen. In contrast to the warm oil, the pack is unheated and is used at room temperature.

INDICATIONS

Abdominal pain, adhesions, appendicitis, colitis, elimination and assimilation problems, food and ptomaine poisoning, gastritis, gland incoordination, inflammation, injuries, intestinal gas, lesions, lymphatic disturbances, pelvic disorders, peritonitis, Recklinghausen's disease, rheumatism, skin cancer, tuberculosis, tumors, typhoid fever, ulcers

MATERIALS NEEDED

Raw, fresh Concord grapes preferred or seedless white grapes; " . . . the larger variety (dark grapes, preferably)." (303-35)—to be mashed, crushed, or " . . . rolled . . . retaining the hull *with* the pulp . . . " (757-6)

Gauze, cheesecloth, or heavy cloth that may be folded or sewn or basted into a bag (like a pillow)—to hold the crushed grapes; cloth placed on top and bottom with grapes in between

Towel or heavy cloth—to be placed over the whole poultice

Flat tray or plate (optional)—on which to set the poultice before applying to the abdomen

FREQUENCY OF APPLICATION

Once or twice daily, 2 days, 3 to 5 days in succession, once a day for 4 to 5 days, once a week, may change to a fresh poultice when body heat warms the pack

LENGTH OF TIME OF APPLICATION

Until warm from body heat, then replace with fresh poultice; until it is " . . . almost dried on the body . . . " (5280-1); 1 to 1½ hours; several hours; 1½ to 5 hours; change every hour or every 2 to 2½ hours; apply for 8, 9, or 12 hours (includes changes of fresh poultice); keep up applications until condition is relieved; until relief is obtained

LOCATION OF APPLICATION

Abdominal area; may include breast area for tumors (683-3)

SIZE OF PACK

One-fourth inch to ½ inch thick, 1 inch thick, 4 inches thick, large enough to cover abdomen

EXPECTED EFFECTS/PURPOSES

Dissipates inflammation
Overcomes nausea
Relieves head and throat irritations
Prevents congestion

Reduces temperature
Strengthens the body

DIRECTIONS

After washing the raw Concord grapes, crush them, rolling them by hand—the seeds along with the pulp and skin. They are not to be put in water or heated. Use enough grapes to place across the abdomen from one-fourth inch thick up to four inches thick. Put the grape mass between two pieces of gauze or cheesecloth on a plate or tray. The pack should be large enough to cover the abdomen. Sew or baste the grapes into a bag (like a pillow). You may want to prepare the bag earlier by sewing up three sides of the cloths together and stuffing the crushed grapes into the opened fourth side. Then sew or baste this side, enclosing the grapes securely into a large pack.

Depending upon the condition and length of time using the pack, you may need to make one or several additional poultices if you intend to replace the earlier one after your body heat has dried it.

The grape poultice is then placed over the abdomen. It will be rather cool, so ease it onto your skin, slowly acclimating your body to the temperature. Once in place lay a heavy cloth over the entire pack. Body heat will eventually warm the pack and almost dry it. Then it can be removed and a fresh, new pack applied, if needed.

> . . . let each poultice remain until it has gotten warm—quite warm from the body heat—or more than temperature of the body. Then add a new one, or put a fresh one on. This should not be necessary more than forty-eight hours. They would be changed about every two or two and a half hours. Use fresh grapes, don't use those over again! . . .
>
> 1237-1

Depending upon the body's response, this reapplication might even be done over the course of three to five days in succession, leaving the poultice on for several hours each day.

DIRECTIONS FROM THE READINGS

For an approximately forty-eight-year-old woman with incoordination difficulties between assimilations and eliminations (reading given on June 13, 1934):

> To reduce the temperature, as well as the inflammation through the abdomen and colon specific, we would use Grape Poultices; preferably Concord Grapes. Crush same and put between gauze, at least half an inch thick, with a heavier cloth on top, and apply directly to the abdominal area. Make the Pack sufficiently large to cover the whole area of the colon and abdomen, you see. Let it remain until warm from the body heat, or as hot as the body, see? then change and put on a fresh Pack . . .   313-16

For a forty-eight-year-old woman suffering from colitis (reading given on July 25, 1936):

> Put a poultice of grapes, cool—grapes of any character, preferably Concord but any character, crushed—except those without seed, don't use those—we want those with seed for it's the tartaric acid that we are giving that we want the reaction from. {*Note: Sometimes seedless grapes were recommended. See* Additional Information.} Crush same, place between thin cloths over the abdomen, extending up to the lower end of the stomach, to overcome this nausea and tendency for the reaction to the head and throat and the irritations that arise.   340-34

For a forty-four-year-old male with amoebic dysentery and neurasthenia (reading given on April 16, 1944):

> Once each day, for a period of at least 4 to 5 days in succession, we would apply a Grape Poultice over the abdominal area, including the lower portion of the liver, extending as low as the caecum. Crush the grapes (the pink California grapes, at this particular season) and apply on gauze about a quarter of an inch to half an inch thick. Allow this poultice to remain until the body has absorbed almost all the moisture

from the grapes. Repeat this each day for at least 5 days.   5023-1

TESTIMONIALS/RESULTS

On October 30, 1935, Miss [852], eighteen years old and suffering from colitis, wrote to Edgar Cayce:

> "I want to thank you for your kindness in giving the readings on me, for I was not responding to the doctors' treatment and received relief only when the first grape poultice was applied. From all accounts, the grape poultice has been discussed all over the town . . . Words cannot express adequately my gratitude to you and all the rest, and I can only say that I wish you the best ever in your work. I am feeling so much better now . . . Last night I ate supper at the table for the first time and were Mamma and Daddy, as well as myself, pleased! Today has been just like summer, so I walked for a few minutes on the front porch and walk."   852-10, Report #1

A thirty-three-year-old woman with impaired digestion, incoordination between assimilations and eliminations, and tuberculosis tendencies, wrote on September 25, 1940:

> "When can I have the check reading? I seem to be worse now than any time. The only thing that gave me relief was the grape poultice . . . When I first got the reading I went for two weeks without vomiting any of my food, by using the grape poultice . . . {*Later she had difficulty getting additional grapes and other recommended items, so was delayed in carrying out her reading further.*}"   2320-1, Report #2

The mother [585] of a fourteen-year-old girl [308] wrote this report on April 2, 1939:

> "The next morning after the reading Hugh Lynn Cayce [Edgar Cayce's son] phoned it to me and told us it was typhoid [fever], and I asked my daughter what she wanted to do, follow the reading or go by what the doctor suggested. She chose the reading. This was the first time my

husband openly opposed Mr. Cayce or the readings, but we followed the reading, as chosen by my daughter. I kept all of the doctor's medicine in sight, so that when he came each day he would say, 'She is getting along fine—just keep up the treatment,' but I was following what had been outlined in the reading.

" . . . What really saved her life was the grape poultice, which brought her temperature down to—at first 101° F., but very gradually. She was too weak to raise her hands, and I never saw her so ill. About the third day she started crying, and begged me to please call Mr. Cayce—'Get me a reading—I don't want to die!' I didn't want to get one too soon after the one just given, but I did call in for a check reading at that time."   308-5, Report #3

A phone call from the brother-in-law of a forty-three-year-old woman [977] with adhesions and nervous system incoordination reported:

"There was a wonderful response to the grape poultice. Her eyes are clearer. The family feels very much encouraged . . . " 977-1, Report #1

ADDITIONAL INFORMATION

Although the readings preferred Concord grapes, because " . . . the *seed* in the Concord grapes are those that take away the inflammation the most . . . " (1045-3), substitutes were also noted if the Concord grapes could not be obtained: "the seedless white grapes" (1045-3), " . . . use the purple grapes that may be obtained—as the California Grapes, but *not* the white grapes!" (324-7), " . . . the colored grapes rather than the green . . . " (1970-1), " . . . the larger variety (dark grapes, preferably)." (303-35), or " . . . as near that type as possible . . . " (464-33)

Today over 400,000 tons of Concord grapes are grown in the northern and eastern United States. A native to U.S. soil, the grapes are named for the Massachusetts village where the first of its variety was grown. They contain protein, calcium, phosphorus, vitamin C, and thiamine, and are known for their hardiness and robustness, ripening early to escape the northern frosts.

Though exceptions to the variety of grape can be made, it is important that the seeds be included when the grapes are crushed because of
the tartaric acid in the seeds, according to reading 340-34. Laboratory
studies have shown that grape seeds contain antioxidants, which help
prevent cell damage from free radicals. Grape seed extract, a popular
herbal treatment, has been used for diabetic complications, heart and
blood vessel conditions, cancer prevention, and wound healing, yet
Cayce never mentioned this product in the text of his readings.

In the chapter on "Colitis" in *Physician's Reference Notebook*, Dr. William
McGarey states that a grape poultice "was suggested in many readings
apparently for its effect on the lymph centers and the lymph fluid as a
cleansing type of preparation." (p. 83) Considering that roughly 200 to
350 lymph nodes reside in the abdomen, placing a grape poultice on
that area would certainly provide a therapeutic benefit for many kinds
of abdominal concerns.

OTHER USES FOR GRAPES

Fresh grapes take a prominent place in the readings as part of a
weight-loss diet, whether eaten whole or in juice form. (*See also* the chapter on "Grape Juice.") The Cayce way to deal with obesity emphasizes a
balanced approach with reductions and some elimination of food
groups as part of one's dietary regimen. Whether eating only grapes for
several days as a mono-diet or drinking diluted grape juice thirty minutes before each meal, this fruit has the capacity to help individuals
control their appetites and reduce their desire for sweets.

In answering a question about the healing properties of grapes and
grape juice, Cayce in his waking state wrote that it was his personal
opinion " . . . absorbed from the information . . . " presented in his
readings that grapes are " . . . one of the best healing foods for any
intestinal disorder . . . " (1942-3, Report #5)

Liver Juice

Various different juices derived from specific vegetables, fruits, or meats are mentioned in the readings for their value as a form of medicine or tonic, supporting the popular idea that food has a medicinal benefit in one's healing process. Onions, potato peelings, grapes, beef, and liver are all mentioned as sources of these juices, to be consumed along with and in conjunction with other modalities.

About sixty readings cite various forms of liver: chopped, broiled, extract, pudding, and juice as part of an individual's dietary regimen—nine of which specified liver juice.

Taken as a medicine, liver juice is prepared the same way as beef juice and is indicated for similar conditions (*see* the chapter "Beef Juice"). It, too, is sipped slowly in small quantities throughout the day, may be drunk warm, and may be eaten with Graham or whole wheat crackers.

In the terminology of the readings, Cayce often spoke of liver extract, which in several instances seemed to be equated with liver juice. However, some individuals' letters referred to inoculations of liver extract that they were receiving, which was available at the time. Several readings disapproved of the shots and preferred that

the extract be taken orally. Liver extract products mentioned and recommended in the readings include: Valentine's Liver Extract (with or
without iron), which is a liquid extract of edible mammalian liver approved by the medical profession since 1929 for pernicious anemia, and
Armour's Liver Extract, which was endorsed in a few readings.

Since not very many details are given in the readings as to the preparation of liver juice, the guidelines for beef juice may be followed, as the
two were usually mentioned in close connection to each other. One
reading states: " . . . liver {juice} may be prepared in the same way and
manner {as beef juice}; for liver extract would be most beneficial for the
body, taken in that same way . . . " (2701-1)

INDICATIONS

Anemia (pernicious), as a strengthener for the body, for blood building, general debilitation, Parkinson's disease, recuperation

MATERIALS NEEDED

One-quarter pound to ½ pound of liver; broiled (calf's) liver, fat removed

Knife—to cut meat into cubes and to remove fat

Glass jar or container with cover

Boiler or pan—to fill with water and in which to place glass jar

Cloth or wire rack—to place under glass jar in pan

Small container—to refrigerate the juice

Tongs (optional)—to extract the liver cubes after boiling

Cheesecloth (optional) or strainer—to strain fat globules after cooking

Patapar paper (optional)—to place liver cubes on rather than into
covered glass jar

Some seasoning (not specified)

FREQUENCY OF DOSAGE

Occasionally, rather often, every day, every other day, 3 or 4 times in
the morning and 3 or 4 times in the afternoon, 2 or 3 times a week

AMOUNT OF DOSAGE

Very small quantities; small amounts, sipped slowly; not too much at one time; " . . . all . . . that the body can assimilate, not to make it obnoxious to the body . . . " (2621-1); 2 tablespoons total for the day, sipped ½ teaspoon at a time; 1 tablespoon total for the day, sipped 1 teaspoon at a time, " . . . taking at least a minute to swallow that amount . . . " (2701-1)

EXPECTED EFFECTS/PURPOSES

Builds up blood and body energies
Combats weakness
Strengthens the body forces
Easy for the body to assimilate
Helpful for recuperation

DIRECTIONS

As noted in the introductory information, liver juice may be prepared in the same way as beef juice. (*See also* the chapter on "Beef Juice.") The amount of liver would depend upon how much and how long you intend to take the juice. One reading stated: " . . . There will be enough in a pound to last for two or three days . . . " (461-1)

The meat can be cut into cubes or broiled. If not broiled, then place the cubes in a glass jar that can be covered. Set the jar into a pan or other stove-top container that is deep enough so that the water added to the pot will cover about one-half to three-fourths of the side of the jar. Cover the top of the jar, but do not seal it tightly.

Set the jar on a cloth or wire rack placed on the bottom of the pan to prevent the jar from cracking. Boil the water about two to four hours. (Option: You may instead place the meat in Patapar paper, tie a bow-knot at the top, set the bag in water, and boil the meat. This will preserve the juice.)

The liver juice will build up gradually and accumulate inside the jar during the boiling process. When finished boiling, let it rest to cool off a bit, then strain the juice with cheesecloth or a strainer, removing all traces of fat and pressing the cubes to extract any remaining liquid in the meat. Place the juice in a small container to be refrigerated up to two or three days—or, as with the beef juice, make it fresh every day or every other day. The juice can even be drunk warm.

Like the beef juice, liver juice is taken in small quantities and sipped slowly, several times during the day. (See *Frequency of Dosage* and *Amount of Dosage*.) Seasoning may be added to make it more palatable; crackers may be eaten along with the juice.

If the liver is broiled, several readings indicate that the piece of meat may be chewed to retrieve the juice. The meat would then be discarded afterward.

DIRECTIONS FROM THE READINGS

For a fifty-three-year-old woman with pelvic tumors (reading given on March 4, 1940):

> (Q) As I cannot eat enough to keep my strength, is there anything I can do to increase my weight?
> (A) Keep those things that have been indicated, and these will *give* the strength—the liver and beef juice, not as a drink but as a medicine. And these—the beef juice and the liver extract—would be sipped, and not taken as a drink, but sipped very slowly. The broiled liver, of course, would be masticated very thoroughly.   2025-3

For a fifty-year-old woman with Parkinson's disease (reading given on May 9, 1939):

> Take more of the beef, or especially *liver* extracts, or liver juices—the liver may be broiled and then the juice pressed out in a squeezer. This taken as food is easily assimilated, and the body may quickly gain strength from same for nerve impulses—especially with the other applications.   1838-3

For a four-year-old girl who was partially deaf (reading given on January 18, 1944):

Do give a great deal of liver juice, though in very small doses at a time; not so much the liver itself, but calf's liver broiled and mashed to a pulp, with a great deal of the juices—so don't make it so hard as to remove all of these. Don't put grease with it.   3571-1

TESTIMONIALS/RESULTS

On October 25, 1936, a forty-one-year-old woman suffering from bronchitis, a cold, and laryngitis wrote a letter to Edgar Cayce:

" . . . How thankful I am to the good Lord to have you when we need you! You were kind, indeed, to answer my appeal so promptly and I want you to know how greatly I appreciate your doing so . . .

"The sore throat started a few days before I wired you but, of course, I didn't realize it would be so severe. Went down to Dr. Thompson on Monday and Tuesday but didn't respond {at} all, so said to him, 'I cannot go on like this, as I am feeling miserable, so am going to wire Mr. Cayce.' I did so and must say that I have been improving ever since. Am following all suggestions but must say the liver extract is a terrible dose. I don't mind that, though, because regardless of what it tasted like I would take it if you told me to do so. I knew that my resistance was terribly low, although I did not realize I have been too active, so shall slow down, after I am able to be out . . . "   1100-7, Report #1

A thirty-one-year-old woman, suffering from debilitation, commented on her experience with the juice—no doubt, a fairly common reaction. On June 28, 1939, she wrote to Cayce:

"By the way, I have taken two doses of the liver extract and I can assure you that you were right in saying it was terrible—ahhhhh I can still taste it!!!"   808-10, Report #2

ADDITIONAL INFORMATION

A sixty-eight-year-old woman, Miss [3587], had received a health reading from Cayce on January 23, 1944. Her nurse-friend later sent a letter, addressed to Cayce, asking for clarification of some statements made in the reading, largely regarding the proper application of the suggestions. She wanted to know if an "extract of liver" could be used in place of the broiled liver if the latter became unobtainable. Gladys Davis answered her letter on March 4, 1944:

> " . . . Due to Mr. Cayce's illness, I am, at this late date, attempting to answer your recent letter.
>
> "The broiled calves liver should be given two or three times a week, or as often as the body can obtain it and take it without tiring of it. The readings do not often recommend liver extract, though I suppose this could be used if the fresh liver is unobtainable."   3587-1, Report #4

The fact that the reading was given during the Second World War when certain items were in short supply may be the reason for the concern about unavailability. Liver extracts, some of which were on the market, were advised in a few readings; but, as stated in the introductory information, some individuals' letters mentioned certain extracts that were taken hypodermically, a practice not approved of in the readings.

Massage

Clearly one of the most frequently suggested remedies in the readings, massage (sometimes referred to as a "rub" or "rubdown" by Cayce), might also be the oldest of any of the applications. By instinct, whenever we suffer a painful injury or accident, we automatically place a hand over the site. We touch or rub it, offering a soothing comfort to the afflicted area. Probably even our early cave-dwelling ancestors from the Stone Age did the same. Eons later in the early 1800s a fencing master and gymnast from Stockholm, Sweden, Per Henrik Ling, is credited with formulating a technique based on scientific principles to work the body. His technique was standardized to what has become known as "Swedish massage," a term that was also used in Cayce's readings as a recommendation for treatment.

The word *massage* appears in over 3,000 readings and was frequently used in conjunction with steam and fume baths, colonics, castor oil packs, and osteopathic adjustments. It affects the entire body—the organs, nerves, circulation—as well as glands and muscles. It can be both stimulating and relaxing, helping to rid the body of toxins and fatigue, quieting the nerves, as well as creating a " . . . change of the vibrations . . . to portions of the body . . . " (390-1) By definition, massage is the manipulation of soft tissue in a therapeutic manner, either by hand or with a mechanical or electrical appliance.

If applied by hand, an oil or powder is used as a lubricant to ease the movement of the strokes and, according to the readings, to add nutriment or other healing properties to the skin and body. Cayce sometimes suggested that the oil be poured in a small bowl or cup, fingers dipped into it, and the oil massaged into the skin. Any oil remaining in the bowl after the massage is discarded because it has come in contact directly with the therapist's fingers and indirectly with the client's body.

Once thought of as a luxury for the wealthy, nowadays massage is regarded as an important element of good health. It helps to eliminate trapped toxins that can cause fatigue or contribute to the start of more serious bodily illnesses. In addition, massage strengthens the immune system that in turn aids the body in fighting disease.

MATERIALS NEEDED

Recommendation of or referral to a professional massage therapist (see also *Directions*)

Lubricant to apply on the skin (various oils and formulas recommended in the readings)

Massage table or folding table draped with sheets and towels; pillow underneath knees

Saucer, bowl, or cup to place oil in (optional)

INDICATIONS

Abrasions, arthritis, bunions, constipation, dry skin, fever (massage with grain alcohol to reduce temperature), gradual hearing loss, headaches, insomnia, joint pain, leg cramps or twitching, menopause, muscle contractions and strain, nervousness, night sweats, peeling skin on feet, poor eyesight, post–surgery (with surgeon's approval), pregnancy (avoid during first trimester), stiff neck and joints, stress, swelling (massage above or around swollen area), varicose veins (avoid area if very enlarged or any clots present), weak arches

CONTRAINDICATIONS

No massages in the following cases: acute infectious diseases (colds, flu, etc.); aneurysm (ballooning of artery); edema (from kidney, liver, or heart disease, cancer, toxemia); shortness of breath from heart or lung problems; intoxication; use of illegal drugs; blood clots (thrombosis, varicose veins); severe, uncontrollable high blood pressure; during first trimester of pregnancy

No massage directly on specific areas: open sores, cuts, burns, or wounds; poison ivy or poison oak outbreaks; athlete's foot, impetigo, scabies, fractures; frostbite; acute inflammation; shingles (if oozing); colostomy, ileostomy, ulcers, hernia (avoid abdomen); cancer (avoid area of tumor)

When using the Wet-Cell Appliance: some readings (such as 1853-1) suggest massage immediately following each use of the Appliance; other readings (such as 1598-2) recommend not having a massage during the period of using the Appliance

For post-surgery, wait 6 weeks or longer and get physician's approval

Guideline for contraindications: "When in doubt, refer out"; that is, if a condition is questionable, clients should check with their health care professional before attempting massage, or the therapist may suggest appropriate physicians to confirm approval for bodywork

FREQUENCY OF APPLICATION

Daily; daily for 5 days; once or twice daily; once every 10 days; 3 times a day (for specific locations); every other day; each evening for 2 weeks; 2, 3, or 4 times weekly; once every 2 weeks; every week for 1 month to 6 weeks; 2 weeks daily, leave off for 10 days, then repeat for 2 weeks daily; once a month; 6 to 10 massages, then a colonic

WHEN TO TAKE THE MASSAGE

Evenings; afternoons; mornings; before retiring or resting; following a series of osteopathic adjustments; after a steam/fume bath, an Epsom Salts bath, exercise, or a castor oil pack; post-surgery (with surgeon's approval)

LENGTH OF TIME OF APPLICATION

Five to 10 minutes (localized applications); 15, 20, to 30 minutes up to 90 minutes; ½ to ¾ hour

LOCATION OF APPLICATION

Abdomen (also massage during colonic); across hips and diaphragm; along cerebrospinal system; along sympathetic system more than cerebrospinal system; along sciatic system; along the side muscles under arms; around the mammary glands; away from the head; behind the knees; clavicle, neck, and head; either side of the spine; feet to knees; following the nerves; hands; limbs (arms and legs); lumbar region (small of the back); lower legs; over liver area; scalp; toes, heels, and soles of the feet

EXPECTED EFFECTS/RESULTS

Increases and stimulates superficial circulation (blood and lymph)
Quiets the nerve forces of the body and helps the body to sleep
Reduces tension and strain and relaxes the body
Removes poisons in muscles and strengthens "the muscular forces" (811-3, 903-18)
Prevents instability, incoordination, and fatigue
Reduces swelling
Speeds rehabilitation after surgery
Releases circulation for better eliminations and stimulates kidney activity
Achieves greater elasticity, strength, and better activity for the body
Creates a properly vibrating nerve and blood supply
Retards and prevents scar tissue
Balances the body's mental and spiritual forces
Invigorates the hair and promotes hair growth on scalp
Aids the body in assimilating blood transfusions
Achieves passive exercise

DIRECTIONS

Massage may be performed by a family member, a professional massage therapist, a chiropractor, an osteopath, a nurse, or in cases of localized treatments, by oneself. All these instances are mentioned in the readings; in some cases Cayce stated that a family member or a spouse would be superior to a professional, especially if he or she understands " . . . how to give manipulations or massage along the spine; not necessary to be a doctor at all." (4885-1) Massage may be given by "One that is in attune with that that is being attempted. Anyone—a nurse, or masseur, or osteopath—may do same." (5467-1), or it " . . . may be done by anyone who is patient and persistent . . . " (3117-2) In another reading when the question was asked who should give the massage, this explanation was offered:

> Anyone that understands the anatomical structure of the body, in knowing how to coordinate the sympathetic and cerebrospinal systems in the areas indicated. These are not merely to be punched or pressed, but the ganglia—while very small—are as networks in these various areas. Hence a gentle, circular massage, is needed; using only at times structural portions as leverages, but not ever—of course—bruising structure.   3075-1

The previous excerpt mentions two items noted in other readings: that the strokes along the spine should be done in a circular motion and that the massage should be gentle and never bruise the body.

Because throughout the readings, as with other remedies, the applications are individualized, it would be too difficult to describe how to give a massage treatment that would be suitable for everyone. Dr. Harold J. Reilly, who received referrals from Cayce for treatments and trained therapists who worked at the A.R.E. in Virginia Beach, had a particular and gifted way of working with the body and passed along some of his knowledge and expertise to those who trained under him. Some of this wisdom is outlined in chapter 9 in his book *The Edgar Cayce Handbook for Health Through Drugless Therapy*, which gives a holistic way of applying the principles of massage to help heal others. Following the illustrations and instructions offered in that chapter would certainly be an excellent way to begin the massage process. Also following the explanations as given in specific readings might be valuable and beneficial; an individual's reading might include the focus of the massage, sometimes directions and sequence of flow, plus a specific lubricant to use for the massage. The amount of oil to be used is determined on an individual basis—just what the skin can absorb.

The Cayce/Reilly® technique, taught at A.R.E.'s Cayce/Reilly® School of Massotherapy, is a unique blend of three types of massage: Swedish, osteopathic, and neuropathic. Swedish, generally very stimulating, is primarily a massage of the muscular forces of the body, sometimes preceded by a fume bath and ending with an alcohol rub. As mentioned earlier, it was developed by Per Henrik Ling, MD (1776–1839), and combines soft tissue manipulations with passive joint movements.

Osteopathic massage involves the musculoskeletal system, focusing on relieving impingements on the cerebrospinal system through balancing muscle tension along the spinal column. This technique can be used as preparation and support for structural manipulations. Though ancient in origin, its present-day roots can be traced to Dr. Andrew Taylor ("A.T.") Still (1828–1917), the "Father of Osteopathy."

A neuropathic massage focuses primarily on the nervous system, with the goal of improving circulation and flow of nerve impulses. Developed at the turn of the twentieth century, it emphasizes lymphatic drainage and control of circulation, both crucial processes for a healthy body.

Along with a blend of these three types of massage, the Cayce/Reilly® technique also includes special movements, rotations, and stretches based on the Cayce readings and the work of Dr. Reilly, a physiotherapist mentioned earlier who worked closely with Cayce. Beginning the massage with the left arm allows for an enhanced flow of blood and lymph. Because the left is the body's receptive side and the side of the heart, beginning there relaxes the client more quickly. All movements are done gently and slowly, in fluid motions that incorporate and balance the entire body field. Benefits to the recipient are a relaxed body with reduced stress and anxiety, allowing for a healthier attitude and an enhanced healing process.

This kind of massage also provides vibration to the body's muscles and, unlike other massage techniques, vibrates the glands and some organs as well. Therapists gently tap the pituitary, pineal, thyroid, and thymus glands as part of the massage procedure. During the abdominal massage, strokes are designed to gently vibrate the liver, gall bladder, spleen, pancreas, and descending colon. The colon is never pushed or massaged against the direction of its natural flow. These vibratory movements help to improve liver function, eliminate toxic waste from the body, and greatly assist those who suffer from constipation or a spastic colon.

In addition, the massage provides range of motion (ROM) to limbs and joints. Every move has a purpose, as illustrated by the gentle head and arm rotations and stretches, with special attention given to the joints of the wrists and fingers. There are hip rotations, diagonal stretches for the back, spinal stretches, and manipulations of the ankle joints. All of these are done slowly and gently, and incorporated into the overall procedure.

One of the many unique characteristics of the Cayce/Reilly® method is the spinal pattern technique. In the readings, four different patterns of spinal manipulation were recommended for various people (see the *Additional Information* section). The most frequently mentioned method was adopted into the Cayce/Reilly® massage work. The technique includes a series of close, small, circular movements that begins at the first cervical vertebra (at the base of the skull) and continues all the way down the spine. These movements are not performed on the muscles on either side of the spine but take place in the groove (called the lamina groove) next to the spine.

The benefit of working in the groove and not on the muscles is that these circular massage movements help to coordinate the nervous systems as both the cerebrospinal and autonomic nervous systems are located here. The massage movements balance these two nervous systems, and the balancing, in turn, affects all systems of the body.

According to the readings, the massage is to be done unhurriedly, prayerfully, and with a healing intent, by one who is patient and persistent and who knows both anatomy and physiology. The readings also encouraged recipients to seek out family members to give them massages. Consider this comment in reply to questioning whether an osteopath should administer the massage:

> Not unless you want to spend a lot of money! Let your wife do it—she'll do it a lot better than the osteopath will!   3381-1

DIRECTIONS FROM THE READINGS

For a twenty-four-year-old recently pregnant woman who also asked for help for neuritis in her arm and shoulder (reading given on May 14, 1927); Cayce told her to begin the massages in sixty days:

> (Q) Would it be best that a caesarean operation be performed or birth take its normal manner?
> (A) It will be born under normal conditions. The normal manner, through the correction of conditions for the body, would be the more satisfactory and the better in the outcome of both. See? Those necessary manipulations may be done by the Swede, or the massage that gives the muscles and tissue across the abdomen and in the lower dorsal and lumbar and sacral region. For these need this massage for the better development of ligaments and tissues as have been involved and as will be involved in the condition.   140-15

For a seven-year-old boy with epilepsy (reading given on July 1, 1938):

> And following such applications {*castor oil packs and abdominal massages*}, we would continue to give the gentle suggestions; but also a massage—when the {*Radio-Active*} Appliance is disconnected. This would be better given along the cerebro-spinal system than over the abdomen. This would be with two fingers on either side of the cerebrospinal system; gently pull downward—that is, beginning at the neck—about half an inch; then press gently; slide just a little more and then press along the whole of the cerebrospinal system.   1625-1

This stroke alonside the spine is referred to as nerve compression in the Cayce/Reilly® routine.

For a fifty-four-year-old woman with spinal subluxations, poor eliminations, and acidity (reading given on May 1, 1936):

> We would use the *fume* baths followed by a thorough rubdown with oils and massage that would produce a better coordination in the eliminating forces of the body; these also removing the poisons that make for a tendency in accumulations through the sympathetic and the activities in the superficial circulation.   906-2

For a twelve-year-old girl who suffered an injury at birth that left her mentally challenged (reading given on September 23, 1943):

> This massage should follow a warm sponge bath especially along the spine. In the head and neck area especially should the massage be given, daily, but the whole spinal area. If this will be given by the mother it will be better, and at the same time suggest to the body what is desired of it . . .
>
> . . . If the body goes to sleep during those periods of massage and suggestion, that much the better . . . Those areas, of course, around the base of the brain, around the edge of the face, through the temple, and back of the ears, all should receive special attention. Then all the rest of the massage should be made downward. The area of the coccyx, the lower lumbar, the limbs and knees and ankles and feet, all should have special attention. Do not do this just to hurry through with it, but be persistent, consistent, and do it all as with a prayer, and with the dedicating of self to a service that this body may indeed be the better channel for the manifestations of the glory of the Creative Forces in a physical being.   3236-1

TESTIMONIALS/RESULTS

A middle-aged woman named Carolyn participated in the beginners' five-day massage workshop sponsored in late December by the Cayce/Reilly® School of Massotherapy. On the first day of class she told the participants that she was taking this workshop to help her elderly mother who had become more listless and debilitated to the extent that she eventually was unable to care for herself. Though not too seriously ill, the mother experienced a number of discomforts and had lost interest in activities around her.

Carolyn said that she just *knew* that massage would be good for her mother, and she wanted to help her. After the workshop she gave her mother daily massages, following the basic, abbreviated Cayce/Reilly® routine that she had learned over the five days. After one month of massages the edema in her mother's ankles cleared up completely. Carolyn had incorporated Dr. Reilly's suggestion in his book, *The Edgar Cayce Handbook for Health Through Drugless Therapy*: to petrissage (knead) the legs up and down several times to alleviate swelling. She continued the daily massages for several months, and the improvement in her mother's condition was remarkable. Her mother had more energy, felt better, took more of an interest in life, and was back to living on her own again. Even her mother's friends noticed the amazing changes in her.

Although Carolyn also encouraged her mother to use castor oil packs and take some herbs, she credits the daily massages for her mother's improvement in health. Subsequently, her mother began raving about the benefits of massage to anyone who would listen. She was indeed a changed person.

Carolyn visited Virginia Beach for a short time six months later and reported on her mother's good progress. Though just at the beginner's level of massage training, she achieved excellent results. "It was through being persistent and consistent," she said emphatically of this accomplishment.

Mr. R., an attorney, came to see Dr. Reilly:

> "He had been pretty badly crippled in an explosion—his left leg had been broken and had terrible rips in it; his kneecap had also been broken. He had been told by his doctor that he might always limp and have to use a cane or crutch."

Dr. Reilly suggested daily home massages and offered to teach his son. After eight to ten instructional visits, the father began receiving daily massages from his son. The result? "Mr. R. has recovered 95 percent movement in his leg and has discarded both the crutches and the cane." The father later commented to Dr. Reilly, "You have been the means not only of making it possible for me to walk normally again, but also of promoting and enhancing my relationship with my son." (*The Edgar Cayce Handbook for Health Through Drugless Therapy*, p. 161)

ADDITIONAL INFORMATION

One often-quoted reading on the purpose of massage was given to an eighteen-year-old male on March 14, 1941:

> . . . The "why" of the massage should be considered. Inactivity causes many of those portions along the spine from which impulses are received to the various organs to be lax, or taut, or to allow same to receive greater impulse than others. The massage aids the ganglia to receive impulse from nerve forces as it aids circulation through the various portions of the organism.   2456-4

Another reading, offering this explanation, gives a further description:

> . . . The massage only assists the impulse for activity from the nerve centers and ganglia to be directed in the activities of the functioning portions of the system that are controlled by certain reflexes or certain impulses created in same.
>
> Just as in that where there may be a clogged line or a dammed stream. If there are particles removed, it allows the greater flow of activity.
>
> And these impulses for mental and physical reaction are necessary for the body to coordinate properly. Hence the massage should assist in the impulses being carried from assimilated forces to the activities of the mental, the physical and the spiritual self.   1553-5

The term *ganglia* is used in both of the previous excerpts. These ganglia (singular: *ganglion*) are masses of neurons, or nerve cells, which form a double chain, extending along each side of the spinal column from the base of the brain to the coccyx. They are connected with each other and with the central nervous system by nerve fibers, while the nerves of the sympathetic nervous system, which have their origin between T-1 and L-2, enter the double chain of ganglia alongside the spine. The small, circular massage movements on each side of the spine help to coordinate and balance the two nervous systems (cerebrospinal and autonomic) that are located there.

Another point made in the readings is that traveling great distances to and from one's appointment may not necessarily be beneficial, as described in one woman's reading:

> . . . the exercise and the energies used in going to and from such activities overbalance that as might be had from such; while the massage by an efficient masseuse close by would allow the greater benefit by not having to overtax self going back and forth.   1158-11

In the *Directions* section, mention is made of four spinal massage patterns Cayce describes in his readings. (For a fuller explanation of these patterns plus illustrations see *Edgar Cayce's Massage, Hydrotherapy, and Healing Oils* by Joseph Duggan and Sandra Duggan, RN) The first, most frequent pattern begins at the base of the brain on the right side and moves downward toward the end of the spine. Repeat on the left side. This is the pattern used in the Cayce/Reilly® routine and probably one that would benefit most individuals. In addition to stimulating circulation, it affects the autonomic nervous system for better coordination.

In the second pattern, one moves from the right side of the head downward but only to the solar plexus area, the 9th dorsal, or T-9, about mid-back where the bra strap might be located. Then move from the lower spine or coccyx area upward toward the solar plexus. Repeat on the left side. Primarily this massage helps promote drainage, releasing congestion in the nerve centers and plexuses.

The third pattern goes slightly opposite pattern number two. It begins in the middle of the back, at the solar plexus area or T-9, and proceeds up toward the head and out the arms; it then starts again at mid-back, going down the spine and out the legs. This massage stimulates nerve impulses of the autonomic and cerebrospinal nervous systems as well as the nerve fibers and helps them coordinate and carry their messages more easily. According to Joseph Duggan, "there seems to be a relationship between this type of massage and the growth process of the body during and immediately following conception . . . " (p. 81). The massage parallels how a person comes into existence by following the pattern of fetal development and is therefore a kind of rebirthing.

In the fourth and final spinal pattern, one moves up the spine. Very few readings mention this upward direction; most readings recommend a downward movement. The upward movement, from the end of the spine toward the brain, seems restricted to painful, physical symptoms and/or mental distress, producing minimal stimulation to the body.

Regarding the oils to be used, you may choose to follow a particular series of readings specific to your condition and decide on those oils recommended, being mindful of the therapeutic properties that Cayce attributed to these lubricants. As Dr. Reilly states in his book, "Cayce did not always explain his selection of a particular oil or mixture, but where we do find explanations there always seemed to be a therapeutic rationale, rather than caprice or custom." (p. 162)

For further information on this topic *see* the following chapters in this book: "Peanut Oil Massage," "Olive Oil," "Castor Oil Pack," and "Myrrh."

Mullein Stupe

A stupe is a cloth wrung out of hot water, which usually contains an added medicament either to relieve pain or to act as an irritant to stimulate local circulation; it has also been described as medicated water. The cloth is applied externally, supplying moist warmth to sores, lesions, or inflamed areas. In the case of mullein, the leaves are soaked in boiling water, placed in layers between gauze, and the moist gauze is then applied to the body.

At least five species of mullein (pronounced mull–in) grow wild in the U.S., though all have been naturalized from Europe. In the summer the plant is easily recognizable due to its velvety, broad, lance-shaped leaves and golden yellow flowers on tall spikes. It can reach up to six feet (two meters) in height and grows on open uncultivated land and along roadsides. Over 140 readings mention mullein, most often designating its use as a tea and a stupe or poultice.

INDICATIONS

Abrasions, bladder problems, boils, bruises, cancer, circulation (blood and lymph) problems, dermatitis, dilation of the abdomen, edema, inflammation, injuries, kidney stones, muscle atrophy, pain, phlebitis, Recklinghausen's disease, swelling, varicose veins

MATERIALS NEEDED

Large leaves of the green (not dried) mullein plant—enough leaves for 2 to 4 layers of thickness (fresh leaves are preferred if in season)

Enamel pan or glass bowl (not tin or metal container)—to place leaves in and soak in boiling water)

Water heated to a boil

Gauze—to place, in some cases, between the mullein and the body

Cotton—to lay upon the gauze

Tray (optional)—to lay out gauze upon to receive the leaves

Heavy towel or cloth—to place on top of the leaf compress to hold in heat

Electric heating pad (optional)—to maintain heat

Plastic (optional)—to place between heating pad and leaf compress

Towel or plastic (optional)—to place under the treated area to protect the sheets

Acid antiseptic solution—to clean area after stupe is removed

FREQUENCY OF APPLICATION

Occasionally, once a day, twice a day, every other day, 1 to 3 times a day, each evening for 3 to 4 days, each evening for 2 weeks, once a week, 2 to 3 times a week, 2 to 3 times a month

LENGTH OF TIME OF APPLICATION

One-half hour to 1 hour; 20 to 30 minutes; 30 to 40 minutes; change every 20 minutes, 3 times during the hour, or every 2 hours; 1 to 3 days; use if pain persists; " . . . until there is relief from the . . . pains . . . " (1375–1); after pain has eased, leave off 1 day, on 1 day, off 2 or 3 days; until the stupe becomes cold; take off, rest 1 to 3 days, reapply; until the leaves have dried

LOCATION OF APPLICATION

Abdomen; along the thigh; ankles; back of the neck; base of head; foot; gall duct area; jaw; just below knee where varicose veins are severe; kidneys; knee; liver; lumbar, sacral, and coccyx areas; over the abrasion or injury; over the eyes; shoulder; swollen area; spine; throat; " . . . those areas that are the *sources* from which the limbs receive their circulatory activity, and those portions about the limb to reduce the swelling . . . " (1541–6); " . . . where the contraction in the muscular forces occurs . . . " (760–17)

SIZE OF PACK
Large enough to cover injured or painful area

EXPECTED EFFECTS/PURPOSES
Reduces swelling and excess fluid
Relieves pain and soreness
Rests and relaxes the system
Increases eliminations (in kidney and bladder)
Absorbs " . . . poisons from the body itself . . . " (988–7)
Helps keep alimentary canal working properly
Dissolves and breaks up kidney stones

DIRECTIONS
Fresh mullein leaves, if available, are what the readings preferred. " . . . Use as broad or large leaves as possible . . . " (3287–1) Some people even asked where they could be obtained. " . . . Grows in most fence corners . . . ," Cayce responded to one gentleman (849–5). "Wherever cows graze in Florida or anywhere else, mullein grows. It is one of the mosses that comes from feeding cattle—cows especially." (3287–2)

Gather and wash thoroughly as many large leaves as you need of the green mullein to make two to four layers to cover the specific area of pain, injury, or varicosity. Bruise the leaves, place them in an enamel or glass bowl or pan (not aluminum or tin), and pour boiling water over them. Let stand for ten to twenty minutes. Another reading states that they should " . . . remain in boiling water a few minutes to wilt them thoroughly . . . " (3287–1). If you wish, lay a thin layer of gauze out on a tray to receive the leaves; the gauze should be the size of the pack needed.

When the water has cooled a little but is still warm, dip out the leaves—do not squeeze all the juice out of them—and place them upon the gauze on the tray or directly onto the body. Make two to four layers of the leaves, about one-fourth to one-half inch thick. Then lay a piece of cotton over the leaves and gauze. There should be enough moisture in the leaves to dampen the cotton somewhat. Place coarse, heavy towels or cloths over the cotton " . . . to be sure that the heat is kept close to the body . . . " (360-5) An electric heating pad may be added for this purpose as well. Insert a piece of plastic between the pad and the heavy cloth to protect the heating pad.

Other readings recommend placing the warm mullein leaves directly onto the skin—no gauze needed. The heavy cloths would still be added on top of the leaves to keep the heat in. In response to a question regarding placement of the mullein leaves, Cayce answered: "They may be applied directly {to the body} or between gauze, depending on the severity of the ulcerated area from time to time . . . " (2714-1)

For how often and how long to use the stupe, see *Frequency of Application* and *Length of Time of Application* to note the variety of choices presented. The decision on how often and how long, as usual, depends upon the severity of the condition and the body's response or reaction to the applications.

Regarding the procedure for reapplying the stupes, this question was asked:

> (Q) In changing the Stupes during the hour, should a new Mullein supply be used, or the same supply reheated?
> (A) The same may be reheated, but each day the Mullein should be new; and as this is beginning to show in its growing, use fresh Mullein. Break it, use it with water—not too much water it is put in, but let the Mullein be almost directly on the skin, or only a thin gauze between the skin and the Mullein, you see, so it may be held in place . . .   1355-1

One reading (988-7) advised that after each stupe is removed the area should be cleaned with an acid antiseptic solution. Another reading explained: " . . . after each use (for this tends to draw), sponge off

with the weakened solution of Bichloride; then apply Cuticura Ointment." (1375-3)

DIRECTIONS FROM THE READINGS

For an eighty-three-year-old man suffering from leg edema (swelling) and asthma (reading given on February 24, 1937):

> ... in the preparing of the Mullein Stupes—put the Mullein into luke-
> warm water and let come almost to a boil; not on a fast or hot boil but
> rather a slow fire ... do not wring it too dry but place between a thin
> layer of cotton, so the cotton becomes moist with the fluids as come from
> the Mullein by the Stupes as well as from the wet Mullein itself. And this
> should become, of course, thoroughly heated, thoroughly saturated—
> that is, the Mullein ... should come to a boil and yet allowed to set after
> turned off until it is sufficiently cool to put the hands in same, see?
>
> Then this upon a gauze cloth; that is, the thin layer of cotton, then
> the cotton over same, see, and this applied {*on the limbs and back*}.
> This allows the moisture (not too much of same, but the heat or the
> moisture) to take up the poisons or to act upon the exterior portions of
> the body.
>
> {*A further question to clarify the amount of mullein needed received
> this reply*:} Sufficient of the Mullein, as has been used, to make the
> Stupe sufficiently large to cover the area, see? And as has been given
> in the preparation, put this on in not too cold or not too hot a water,
> just tepid; allowed to come to a boil and then this set aside until cool or
> sufficiently cool to put the hands in same easily, see? Do not squeeze
> all of the juice out of same, for it should be sufficient to dampen the
> cotton that is laid upon the gauze, see? ...   304-45

For a female adult who had previously experienced dental problems
resulting in neck and head pain and who also had poor lymph circulation (reading given on May 28, 1942):

> In the present, then, we would administer the Mullein Stupes to the
> back of neck and shoulders. Use as large leaves as practical. Bruise

them and put in very hot water, letting them stand—or steep—for a few minutes before taking out. Though it may make a messy application, we find that these will be effective. Apply on gauze, {put} cloth over same, and then an electric pad may be applied to keep same warm. This will aid. For, these will add to the system the helpful forces in alleviating pain through head and neck.   2722-4

For a twenty-five-year-old man with Recklinghausen's disease, a genetic disorder involving tumors along various types of nerves as well as bones, muscles, and skin (two doctors were present for this reading given on November 19, 1935):

But to overcome the dropsical or fluid forming portions in the limb and in the abdomen, use the Mullein Stupes—Mullein Stupes. These are to be used at least twice a day. The activities of same upon the body itself will tend to make for the accumulations to be thrown off through the perspiratory system, excessively. Hence it is necessary after each of these stupes that there be used an alkalin or an acid (preferably an acid) antiseptic solution, for the cleansing of the limb and the abdomen. These stupes may be given for a period of half an hour to an hour, so long as they are kept in a manner that they will be active to remove the accumulations.   988-7

For a thirty-one-year-old osteopath who had a variety of diagnoses, for whom eventually the disorder was described as an effect of the nerve system on his liver and kidneys (reading given on May 16, 1939):

Also each evening—and *early* morning—that is, in the evening before retiring, and at the early morning period when the body becomes restless by the sediments that tend to gather in the kidney and bladder, and the irritation that comes from same—we would apply the Green (if possible to obtain) Mullein Stupes. These should be applied over both the liver and gall duct area, and over the kidney area from the back. These should remain upon the body for at least twenty to thirty minutes to an hour, depending upon the ease that same brings, to be sure. In making the Stupes—let these be prepared with the *Green*

Mullein if possible—this bruised and then the hot water poured on same (in a crock or enamel container). Have them at least two thicknesses over the body, with a gauze and then heavy padding afterward—and even an electric pad over both areas would be beneficial. 1885-1

TESTIMONIALS/RESULTS

In the follow-up reports some recipients had difficulty obtaining fresh mullein; one company's name was supplied to them as a source of mullein: S.B. Penick & Company in Asheville, North Carolina. Others had rashes or adverse reactions to the stupes; some complained of the difficulty of making the pack. A forty-nine-year-old bookkeeper, cook, and housekeeper had received two readings from Cayce in 1943—a life reading and a physical reading. On October 29, 1948, a few years after Cayce's death, she wrote:

> "I found the mullein leaves most helpful for varicose veins . . . Also several of our friends who suffered from this malady have been helped. I was about to have my legs operated on last spring when I read the extract from Edgar Cayce's reading 243-38. I found relief and do not now find cause for surgery. Mr. Cayce is still helping me when need arises . . . "   243-38, Report #3

For the twenty-five-year-old man with Recklinghausen's disease (see *Directions from the Readings*) this report was submitted by Dr. John R. Thompson in a letter dated December 23, 1935:

> "[988] seems to be doing very nicely. The swelling of the leg is responding wonderfully to the mullein packs, he can be rolled around easily now and it used to be that the slightest move caused him a great amount of pain. As for the pain, it persists, but doesn't seem to me to have the severity that it used to—at least the effects aren't so great . . . "   988-11, Report #1

ADDITIONAL INFORMATION

An old superstition claims that witches used mullein wicks in their candles and lamps when making incantations; hence, the herb is sometimes called "hag's taper," one of its many appellations. Other names include Common mullein, flannel plant, velvet or mullein dock, candlewick, Aaron's rod, lungwort, and velvet plant. Its power to drive away evil spirits was well known throughout Europe and Asia, demonstrated by Ulysses who used it to protect himself against the wiles of Circe. Mullein's versatile array of uses, according to the recommendations from the Cayce readings, may make this herb seem like a magic potion.

Several readings mention the distinction between using the dry versus the green mullein.

> ... Only the green Mullein would be applied in the stupes, though the dried Mullein may be used in the tea. Of course, the green may also be used for the tea, though it doesn't require so much—about half the quantity—but do not let it boil; just steep as tea, by pouring hot water over same. Let it stand for fifteen or twenty minutes, see?   2714-1

Regarding the same topic a rather humorous question–and–answer exchange took place:

> (Q) Does it make any difference whether the Mullein is dried or fresh?
> (A) Does it make any difference whether cabbage is wilted before it is boiled? It should indeed be fresh, not as in people, but as in the vegetable kingdom; not applying to people being fresh, but plants used for medicinal purposes, the fresher, the more active the better. And there is quite a variation between green Mullein and dried Mullein, but whichever you use, use the same all the while.   457-14

OTHER USES FOR MULLEIN

Besides using mullein stupes for certain conditions, drinking a cup of mullein tea is also advised, using either the fresh or dried leaves. External applications of the tea, mentioned in two readings, are recommended for bathing the skin and washing the hands. More explanation is contained in the chapter "Mullein Tea."

Mullein Tea

This herb has been used since ancient times in folk medicine, largely for respiratory ailments. Mullein tea, made from its yellow flowers, has been used as a remedy for sore throats and coughs and also as a gargle. In the Cayce readings, the leaves, flowers, and/or seeds are steeped in boiling water and the beverage is drunk as a tea. It is sometimes taken in conjunction with mullein stupes, particularly in the case of varicose veins.

Gladys Davis sent Mrs. [1541] the directions for preparing mullein tea, explaining that these same instructions were given in another reading, "so I'm sure they wouldn't hurt here":

> "Take 2 ounces of the Mullein Leaves and bruise very thoroughly, if the green leaves are used, or 3 ounces of the Mullein Leaves if the dried leaves are used, and put into a quart of nearly cold water. Let it come to almost a boil, but very slowly. As it comes to the boil, take off . . . "
> 1541-6, Report #1

The tea is to be kept in a cool place and made fresh every two or three days.

One reading stated: " . . . {*mullein tea*} taken occasionally is not bad for anybody . . . " (457-14)

INDICATIONS
Circulation (blood and lymph) problems, dizziness, hives, intestinal inflammation, kidney stones, varicose veins

MATERIALS NEEDED
Dried or crumbled mullein leaves, flowers, and/or seeds—various amounts from 1 pinch up to 6 ounces

Enamel pan or glass bowl (not aluminum, tin, or metal)—in which to place leaves and add the boiling water

Boiling water—various amounts from 2 ounces up to 1 quart

FREQUENCY OF DOSAGE
During the day, daily, each morning before breakfast, evenings, once or twice daily, several times a day, every other day, once a week, 3 times a week

AMOUNT OF DOSAGE
One teaspoon; ½ ounce; 1, 1½, or 2 ounces; ⅔ teacup; 1 teacup; 1 quart during the day; *ratio of amount of mullein (fresh or dried) to amount of water:* 1 or 2 pinches of dried mullein: 1 cup of water; 1 level teaspoon (flowers): 1 pint water; 1 tablespoon (dried): 2 ounces water; 1 tablespoon (flowers and seeds): 1 pint water; ½ dram (flowers): 1 quart water; 1 dram [¹⁄₁₆ of an ounce] (fresh leaves): 1 pint water; 1 ounce (fresh leaves): 1 pint water; 2 ounces (fresh leaves and/or flowers): 1 quart water; 2 ounces (by weight): 1 pint water; 3 ounces (dried): 1 quart water; 1 teacupful (seeds or blossoms): 1 quart water; 6 ounces: 1 pint water

WHEN TO TAKE THE MULLEIN TEA
Before breakfast, before retiring, evenings

EXPECTED EFFECTS/PURPOSES
Aids in coordinating the circulation

Eliminates acids and poisons from the system

Helps " . . . the general condition of the inflammation throughout the intestinal system." (1375-3)

Cleanses liver and kidneys

Makes for better eliminations

Reduces " . . . accumulation of lymph through the abdomen and the limbs . . . " (409-36)

Relieves pressure upon the kidneys and helps to expel stones

Helps with dizziness

Can be drunk on alternate days with mullein stupes (for relief of varicose veins)

DIRECTIONS

Wash the leaves, seeds, and/or flowers of the fresh mullein plant thoroughly before boiling them for tea. The leaves are cut, bruised, or crushed, and then boiling water is poured over them. Dried mullein may also be used, in which case—according to reading 2714-1—the quantity of the dried mullein would be about twice as much as using the green mullein. In either case—fresh or dried—boiling water is poured over the mullein, and the mixture then is either steeped as a tea or allowed to simmer (but not boil). The steeping and boiling should be done in an enamel or a glass container. The mixture is covered during the steeping.

Strain the tea through cheesecloth or gauze. When it is cool, drink a small amount, ranging from one or two ounces up to a teacup, at a time (see *Amount of Dosage*, which also contains information on how much mullein to use in proportion to the amount of boiling water). The tea is to be refrigerated and made fresh every two or three days.

DIRECTIONS FROM THE READINGS

For a forty-year-old waitress whose doctors could not determine whether she had athlete's foot or eczema in addition to her swollen feet and inability to work (reading given on August 27, 1940):

Each day—preferably just before retiring—take internally about an ounce or ounce and a half of Mullein Tea. Prepare same in this manner; preferably gathering the Mullein Leaves *and* the flower fresh—at this season: Cut these very fine, and put about two ounces of same (by measure, not by weight) in a quart of water. Let this steep as tea. Do not attempt to keep this longer than two days, even with keeping same on ice, for it will not keep, you see. Hence it should be made fresh every third day, you see.   2332-1

For a thirteen–year–old girl suffering from aching legs and trench mouth whose condition was attributed by Cayce to an " . . . infectious condition in the lymph circulation . . . " (reading given on April 1, 1942):

Also once each day, in the evening, take two ounces of Mullein Tea, preferably made from the fresh leaves, see? Cut, bruise or crush the Mullein leaves, and pour a pint of boiling water over a heaping tablespoonful of the crushed leaves and allow to steep as tea—for fifteen to twenty minutes; covered, of course, during the time, and use only a glass or enamel container for boiling the water and for steeping same.
                                                                          2715-1

For a forty–eight–year–old woman with varicose veins (reading given on April 19, 1944):

Take internally each day about two-thirds of a teacup of Mullein Tea. Use dried mullein for this—a pinch between thumb and forefinger, put in a cup and pour boiling water over same, allowing to set for thirty minutes. Strain off, cool and drink just about two-thirds of a cup, daily.
                                                                          5037-1

TESTIMONIALS/RESULTS

Not much follow–up information regarding mullein tea exists in the files. On June 27, 1972, Mrs. Byron Moreland from Minneapolis, Minnesota, wrote to the A.R.E.:

"My husband had a blood clot on his ankle (thrombo-phlebitis). He took only one of the pills his doctor prescribed and then began using Mullein tea as Cayce prescribed. His blood clot disappeared in a very short time. I have a small garden in my back yard and among my lettuce and carrots I have some nice healthy Mullein plants which I am carefully nurturing! I dry some of the leaves periodically for winter use."   5089-4, Report #8

On August 27, 1940, Edgar Cayce wrote a letter to Mrs. [2102] recommending mullein tea for hives:

" . . . Sorry to hear you are still having trouble with the hives—must be something in your diet . . . would suggest, Mrs. [2102], that you go out on the island there somewhere and get you some [mullein] . . . think if you will make you a tea of this, use some of the flower, say take about two ounces—and put in a quart of water, bruise the leaves or cut them up—and steep like tea. Take about two ounces of the tea each day, think you will get rid of the trouble."   2102-3, Report #8

No information exists as to whether or not she followed his suggestion. She had no further readings.

ADDITIONAL INFORMATION

Mullein (botanical name, *Verbascum thapsus*), a biennial plant, is common in the U.S. but undoubtedly introduced from Europe. Growing along roadsides, in open fields, and in recent clearings, it is easily recognized for its straight and tall stem, its hairy, lance-shaped leaves, and the golden-yellow flowers that bloom from June to August. It has been used for coughs, congestion, bronchitis, and for the reduction of mucous formation.

In applying the combination of mullein stupes and tea for one female adult, the reading presented an additional beneficial effect for this remedy: it would " . . . *enable* the body to keep away from the sedatives. But do not overtax the system. Use a hypnotic rather than a narcotic as the sedative. These as we find would be the better." (2722-4)

She had been taking pain pills on a regular basis.

Regarding the freshness of the tea in addition to making a new batch every two or three days, a two-year-old infant boy was advised to take a teaspoonful of the tea two or three times daily; then a caution was added: " . . . Be mindful that this does not sour, or become discolored or get sufficiently heated for it to form any skim over the top." (1990-4)

OTHER USES FOR MULLEIN TEA

For severe itching on the hands this suggestion to an adult male with dermatitis was offered during his second reading on April 24, 1937:

> . . . we would keep the Sweet Oil {*olive oil*} on the hands—preferably, or especially, after they have been bathed or washed in a strong solution of tea from the Mullein Leaves. The hands should be rubbed off in this tea, you see, just as if washing the hands. Then when they are dried (by sponging with the towel, rather than rubbing), pat or rub on the Sweet Oil. This will relieve the tension and the pressure.   1358-2

A twenty-eight-year-old man was offered similar information in his seventeenth reading on March 21, 1937—the use of mullein tea as a hand rinse for his eczema:

> About once a day rinse the hands well in a Mullein Tea. It is preferable (as this is the season it may be had) to use the fresh Mullein. Take two ounces of the Mullein, bruise it very thoroughly and put in nearly cold water and let it come to almost a boil, but very slowly. As it comes to the boil take off. Use this for about two days, then make fresh. Put the two ounces into a quart of water.   1005-17

A sixty-three-year-old male teacher was given this advice for his eczema:

> Of course, rubs or massages will be helpful. Bathing the affected portions of the skin itself with a very heavy or strong tea made from Mullein Leaves would be most helpful. Take two ounces of the Mullein Leaves and bruise very thoroughly, if the green leaves are used, or

three ounces of the Mullein Leaves if the dried leaves are used, and put into a quart of nearly cold water. Let it come to almost a boil, but very slowly. As it comes to the boil take off. Use this proportion in preparing same, for use in bathing the affected parts, but make fresh every two days. This would be a most efficacious application.   1383-1

Besides its use as a tea, in the Cayce readings mullein is also recommended as a stupe. For the mullein stupe, the fresh leaves are placed in a cloth compress and applied to the body for various conditions, especially for varicose veins. *See* the chapter titled "Mullein Stupe" for more information on this use.

Considering its beneficial purposes, mullein—as a tea or stupe—can provide relief for a number of ailments.

Myrrh

Mentioned in nearly four hundred Cayce readings, myrrh, applied externally as an ingredient in a massage formula, is more properly called "tincture of myrrh." (A tincture means that the substance is an alcoholic solution of the herb.) Most often it is used in equal parts with olive oil; in a few instances, sassafras oil or compound tincture of benzoin is added as well. Additionally, myrrh is listed as an ingredient in several tonics, pellets, inhalants, and other massage lotions, for douches and sitz baths, to remove residue from the eyes after a potato poultice, and as an additive in a steam bath.

INDICATIONS

(For massages) Bedsores, calluses, cramping of hands and feet, cysts, fatigue, hernia, itching on abdomen, lumbar strain, muscle soreness, poor assimilations, poor eliminations, spinal subluxations, strains, tender skin (on back), tension, tumors

(In douches and sitz baths) Attempting conception, gynecological problems, itching, pruritus vulvae, vaginitis (*see also* the chapter on "Sitz Bath"), weak uterine walls

(In pellets) Debilitation

(In steam/fume baths) Itching, poor eliminations, tension

(Tonics) Dysmenorrhea, neurosis, pelvic cellulitis, poor eliminations

MATERIALS NEEDED

Bottle of tincture of myrrh

Bottle of pure, extra virgin olive oil (often used in equal parts with myrrh in massages)

Basin of warm water—large enough to hold 1½ gallons of water (for sitz baths)

Baking soda (1 teaspoon) and warm water (1 pint)—to clean area after abdominal massage (optional)

Bowl, saucer, or cup—to place mixture in (optional)

Grain alcohol—to apply as a rubdown after the massage (optional)

FREQUENCY OF APPLICATION

(Massages) Occasionally; once or twice a day; each evening; every other day; 1, 2, or 3 times a week

(Douches) Once a day, once every 3 days, just before menses

(Sitz baths) Once a day, every second or third day, before menses, after menses (see also *Amount of Dosage*)

AMOUNT OF DOSAGE

(Massages: myrrh plus olive oil) Two teaspoons each, 2 tablespoons each, what the body will absorb

(Douches) Two drops tincture of myrrh, 2 drops balsam of Tolu (2457-1); to 1 gallon soft water, add 10 drops Glyco-Thymoline and 3 drops tincture of myrrh, use 2 times just before menses (2722-2); to ½ gallon of soft water at 70°F (21.1°C), add 5 drops Peruvian balsam (also known as balsam of Tolu) plus 5 drops tincture of myrrh (4094-1)

(Sitz baths) To 1½ gallons of very warm water, add 5 drops tincture of myrrh plus 10 grains balsam of Tolu in a basin (538-8); place 1 aloe and 20 drops tincture of myrrh into boiling water—sit over it (222-1); to ½ gallon hot or boiling water, add 1 aloe, 5 drops tincture of myrrh, 40 drops tolu in solution (or balsam Tolu) (5671-6); to 1½ gallons very hot water, add 2 drams gum of balsam of Myrrh—sit over the fumes (199-1);

to 1 gallon steaming, hot water, add 1 teaspoon tincture of myrrh plus 1 teaspoon tolu in solution—sit over it every third day for 20 to 30 minutes (302-8); to 1½ to 2 gallons hot, nearly boiling water, add 15 grains sweet gum plus 1 tablespoon tincture of myrrh—sit over it once a day for 3 to 5 days after menses (2720-2); to 1½ gallons very hot water, add 1 ounce tincture of myrrh plus 30 grains balsam of Tolu (for conception)—sit over it (3980-1); to 1½ gallons very hot water or boiling water, add 20 drops tincture of myrrh plus 20 drops tincture of sweet gum—sit over it for 15 to 20 minutes once each day (4890-1); to 2 gallons very hot water, add ½ teaspoon tincture of myrrh plus ½ teaspoon tolu in solution—sit over it before menses (219-3)

(After potato poultices) Bathe eye with 10% solution of boric acid and 10% solution of tincture of myrrh (3884-1)

(Tonics) Include 20 minims tincture of myrrh with other ingredients—take 2 teaspoons before each meal, for neurosis and poor eliminations (4133-2); include 5 minims tincture of myrrh with other ingredients—take 2 teaspoons 4 times a day after meals, for pelvic cellulitis and dysmenorrhea (5700-2)

(Pellets) Include 36 grains myrrh with other ingredients, makes 24 pellets—take one a day, for blood-building and " . . . to create the appetite necessary to rebuild the system." (4542-1)

(Inhalant) Include 5 minims balsam of myrrh plus other ingredients—small amount poured into receptacle and heated; inhale fumes (4790-1)

(Bath) For rash, bathe parts of skin where rash is located; use 20% boric acid wash plus 10% tincture of myrrh—once a day (5473-3)

WHEN TO TAKE THE MYRRH AND OLIVE OIL

After a castor oil pack, after a dry heat cabinet sweat bath, following an osteopathic manipulation, morning or evening, after or during a massage (apply myrrh and olive oil mixture locally), in the morning following a bath

LENGTH OF TIME OF APPLICATION

(Massages) Two to 3 minutes, 20 to 30 to 40 to 50 minutes

(Douches) Twice a week, 2 times just before menses

(Sitz baths) Two to 10 minutes [begin with 2 minutes, on third day 3 minutes, etc., gradually increasing time limit (5671-6)]; every third day for 20 to 30 minutes

LOCATION OF APPLICATION

Abdomen, about the neck, along length of cerebrospinal system, along the spine, between eyes and the nerves of the face, down the centers of the nerves, feet, fingertips, hips, jaw, ligaments along the spine, the limbs, lower abdomen, lower back, scar tissue, shin bone, shoulders, thyroid region, under the arms, under the side, where the castor oil packs have been applied, whole body

EXPECTED EFFECTS/PURPOSES

Acts with the pores of the skin " . . . to strike in, causing the circulation to be carried to affected parts . . . " (440-3)

Relieves tension and strain and allows the muscles to relax more

Increases stimulation and stimulates the glands

Strengthens the muscles and the body

Provides food value, stability, and strength to the blood capillaries

Equalizes nerve tension and circulation throughout the body

Aids in capillary and lymph circulation

Assists in proper eliminations and in bringing normal conditions to the digestion

Makes " . . . for a better respiratory activity . . . " (626-1)

Prevents the body from being sore in areas of application (such as the back)

Acts " . . . as an absorbent for information along the intestinal area, or as a counter-irritant . . . " (1331-1)

DIRECTIONS

The combination of equal parts tincture of myrrh and olive oil is mixed by heating the oil, then adding the myrrh, and stirring it in. If the oil is not heated, the two substances remain separate and do not blend as they should. Make just the amount you will need for the application;

therefore, the combination is made fresh with each use.

How hot do you warm the oil? One reading says, " . . . not to boiling—but nearly so . . . " (5467-1), before you add the myrrh. Not a great quantity needs to be made, as stated earlier, since most often only a small area or areas would receive the application. Of course, you would put it on right away after mixing it because later, when it begins to cool, it will separate. Shake the mixture before using it.

Only one reading advised the opposite; that is, to heat the *myrrh*, then add the oil. The explanation given is that " . . . this will make for more of an ointment (while the other would remain in a different solution entirely)." (4873-1)

Evidently these two substances act as a team, the myrrh is a carrier (one reading states that the oil is a carrier), while the oil acts as a food and a stimulant, creating a proper lubricant that is carried into the capillary circulation—according to reading 4382-4.

A rubdown with grain alcohol after the olive oil and myrrh massage is suggested in a few readings.

DIRECTIONS FROM THE READINGS

For a sixty-four-year-old woman suffering from apoplexy, hypertension, and a prolapsed colon (reading given on November 13, 1937):

> (Q) {*What causes*} the cramping of hands and feet?
> (A) This is from pressures upon the nerve system, as indicated.
>   When the massage is given with the Olive Oil and Myrrh, heat the oil to add the myrrh, and massage not only along the spine but around the limbs as well as down the centers of the nerves to same; under the arms, you see, along the whole length of the arm, under side, following the nerves to the fingertips—as well as the limbs themselves to the feet; removing the pressures. This is so the circulation may be released for better eliminations.   618-4

For an adult woman with pelvic disorders and problems with sterility (reading given on September 4, 1924):

To a gallon and a half of very hot water in a pail, or container over which the body may sit, add one ounce of Tincture of Myrrh, and 30 grains of Balsam of Tolu. Let this be covered until Tolu is dissolved. Then let the body sit over this and the steam from same enter the pubes and to the parts of body. This will add to the incentive to produce in the system the conditions necessary to bring about conception. This we will find can be completed within four to six months. Not necessary that this be used continually, but use consistently with the conditions ... Do that for these conditions, and we will find that the first child will be a girl that will be born to this body, [3980].   3980-1

[In early 1926, following a doctor's examination, she was told that she was pregnant. A few months later, however, she wrote to Edgar Cayce to tell him she wasn't. No further information is available about this situation.]

For an adult woman with pelvic disorders and lumbago (reading given on October 12, 1922):

We would use as a solution to strengthen the forces through the vagina here this as a douche, and this should be used at the regular periods, and intervals necessary to bring the normal functioning of organs of the pelvis, that is, the ovarian discharge and the discharge from the uterus here, you see. This we would use as a douche. To one gallon of soft water we would add ten drops of glyco-thymoline, with three drops of myrrh. This will only be used twice just before, that is, a day apart for the period you see, when the discharges, see?   2722-2

TESTIMONIALS/RESULTS
Miss [283], who was forty–six years old at the time of her reading, had a large tumor in her abdomen and sent a letter to Edgar Cayce dated October 29, 1927:

" . . . I had a reading from you on July 22, 1927, in regard to my bodily conditions. In it you said that after 30-60 days' treatment as directed I should report further directions and treatment, which is the purpose of this letter.

"First of all I wish to thank you for your diagnosis and treatment and tell you how much it has done for me. I have been greatly helped and benefited by the treatment so far, and with your assurance that cases like mine have been cured, am sure that I also can be *entirely* relieved.

"I had the rubbings in the pelvic and lumbar regions and the spine with olive oil and myrrh as directed, which brought a great deal relief from nervous irritation . . . "   283-1, Report #3

Mrs. [2072] wrote a summary of her condition to Hugh Lynn Cayce on August 16, 1958. Her reading, 2072-16, was given on May 22, 1944, when she was thirty-four years old and had problems with assimilation and elimination as well as spinal subluxations. Her letter reads in part:

" . . . I have used peanut oil rubs, and Olive Oil and Tincture of Myrrh rubs almost every night for a long, long time. Shall keep them up because I know them to be good, and because many of my habits have been based on your father's readings . . . "   2072-16, Report #31

A number of respondents mentioned breaking out with skin irritations and rashes after the olive oil and myrrh massage, attributing these irritations largely to the effects of the myrrh. Some omitted this treatment altogether, others resumed it later with no ill effects. Several others reported that they were receiving the massages, but did not note the results. It was reported that even Gertrude Cayce, Edgar's wife, several weeks before her death was receiving a spinal rub with olive oil and myrrh " . . . to rest and relax her . . . " (538-71, Report #17)

ADDITIONAL INFORMATION

The following is a recipe from the readings using myrrh for a sometimes difficult-to-treat ailment:

(Q) What can be done to relieve bed soreness?

(A) Equal portions of Olive Oil, Tincture of Myrrh and Tincture—Compound Tincture of Benzoin. Heat the Olive Oil to add the other ingredients, in the order named. Massage same or rub on, gently. This should make for such a stimulation in the superficial circulation—where there is the soreness or tenderness formed by the continual pressure in the areas where the body rests upon the bed—as to be more in accord with that which allows normal activity.

Use this once, twice or more during a day, and it should be the more helpful for the body.   988-9

Myrrh is a reddish-brown resin or gum that originates from a bush native to East Africa and Arabia, where over 135 species are found. Growing mainly in arid regions, it is mentioned in both the Old and New Testaments. The Christmas carol "We Three Kings of Orient Are" alludes to its use with these words: "Myrrh is mine, its bitter perfume/ breathes a life of gathering gloom/ . . . sealed in the stone-cold tomb." Myrrh was used not only as a perfume in which the gum was pressed into cakes but also as a salve for purifying the dead, as a spice, and as incense. An effective antimicrobial agent, it is used to treat gum, mouth, and catarrhal problems such as mouth sores, toothache, ulcerated throat, and sinusitis, and as a liniment for bruises, abrasions, aches, and sprains.

As noted previously, myrrh's association with one of the gifts from the Three Kings, Magi, or Wise Men to the infant Jesus is familiar to most people, and its significance has long been open to speculation. In one reading, Cayce elaborated on the symbolism of each of the three gifts: " . . . they represent in the metaphysical sense the three phases of man's experience in materiality; gold, the material; frankincense, the ether or ethereal; myrrh, the healing force . . . " (5749-7) Perhaps this healing force can be kept in mind when one is applying or using this herb for relief and strength.

Olive Oil

Like both castor oil and peanut oil, olive oil has many beneficial effects and multiple uses, some of which may be surprising. It is one of the most frequently mentioned oils, occurring in nearly 1,400 readings. Aside from its common usage as a dressing for salads or as a lubricant for massages, the oil is to be taken after completing the three-day apple diet, following a series of castor oil packs. In some instances, olive oil is recommended for use as a laxative, for a flannel cloth pack, in an enema, as an ingredient in a shampoo, and as an additive in a steam/fume bath.

INDICATIONS

(Laxative) Acidity, constipation, poor digestion, poor eliminations

(Massage) Asthenia, dry skin, hearing difficulties, impaired locomotion, itchy scalp (local), toxemia

(Packs—four cases) Cold and fever, colitis (two cases), relaxation prior to osteopathic adjustments

(Fume bath—one case) Toxemia (olive oil and witch hazel)

CONTRAINDICATIONS

Caution: If one has a history of gallbladder trouble or a liver condition—take orally the minimum amount of olive oil

MATERIALS NEEDED

Bottle of pure olive oil
Flannel cloth (if using the oil in a pack)
Massage table or folding table draped with sheets and towels (if using the oil as a lubricant)
Bowl, saucer, or cup (to place oil in for massage)
Measuring cup or spoon

FREQUENCY OF APPLICATION

(Laxative) Every hour; every few hours; 2 to 3 to 4 hours apart; every 2 hours during the afternoon; 4 to 5 times a day; 2 to 3 days every 2 to 3 hours, leave off 2 to 3 days; 4 to 10 to 40 times a day

(Pack) Change every 20 to 25 minutes

(After a castor oil pack) One time only, often, 3 or 4 times a day, once a week (see also *Amount of Dosage of Olive Oil* in the chapter on "Castor Oil Pack")

(Massage) Once a day, 2 to 3 times a week, once a week, once every 10 days

AMOUNT OF DOSAGE

(Laxative) Small doses; a few drops or sips; ¼, ⅓, ½ teaspoon up to 2 teaspoons; no more than what one's body can assimilate

(Enema) One-half pint

(After a castor oil pack) Very small quantities; ¼ teaspoon up to half a teacup (1 teacup equals about 3 to 8 fluid ounces) [only a few readings mention taking the olive oil on the same days as the packs] (see also *Amount of Dosage of Olive Oil* in the chapter on "Castor Oil Pack")

(On salads) One teaspoonful

(After 3-day apple diet) Half a teacup, half a cup (see also *Amount of Dosage* in chapter on "Apple Diet")

(Massage) One to 2 tablespoons

WHEN TO TAKE THE OLIVE OIL

For any intestinal disturbance; " . . . preferably before meals . . . " (337–1); after completion of a series of castor oil packs (only a few readings mention taking the olive oil on the same days as the packs); on the last day of the 3–day apple diet [the apples plus the olive oil " . . . will cleanse *all* toxic forces from any system! . . . " (820–2)]

LENGTH OF TIME OF APPLICATION

(Laxative) Two to 3 days, 3 to 5 days, 1 week to 10 days, " . . . until there is good evacuation from the alimentary canal . . . " (5146–1)

(Pack) Until a reaction is produced in the liver

(After a castor oil pack) One to 2 months, " . . . until there are the eliminations . . . " (3670–1)

LOCATION OF APPLICATION

(Pack) Across the intestine and lower bowel; areas on back that need relaxation (pack with equal amounts of olive and peanut oil); lower end of stomach, liver, on right side (spirits of camphor added to olive oil); on abdomen and side; right side, ascending colon

(Massage) All over the body; along the spine; arm pits, elbows, groin, knees, temples (lymph centers); knees, hips, abdomen, shoulders, head and neck (with equal amounts of olive oil and tincture of myrrh); limbs; lower portion of lumbar and sacral areas

EXPECTED EFFECTS/PURPOSES

Stimulates muscular and mucus–membrane activity (massage)

Purifies and drains the colon and gall duct (after castor oil pack)

Assists the peristaltic movement of the colon and acts " . . . as a lubricant and as a food for the digestive system . . . " (257–13) (laxative)

Helps eliminate poisons and accumulations and cleanses the alimentary canal (after castor oil pack)

Gives " . . . proper toning of the digestive system . . . " (2092–1) (on salads)

Relieves pressure and irritation from the kidneys and bladder, and distress " . . . in the muscular forces in the descending colon." (340–7) (in enema)

Helps stimulate the walls of the intestinal tract by increasing circulation (pack)

Is food for the skin, tissue, and muscles of the body (massage)

DIRECTIONS

In the Cayce readings olive oil, taken orally, is a **laxative** from which
anyone may benefit. Just how to take it varies slightly from reading to
reading, yet this typical excerpt describes one way as well as emphasizes the readings' principle of consistency:

> Be well for everybody to take olive oil . . . taken occasionally, that is
> consistently—two or three days, and then leave it off. Don't take it one
> day with only one dose and then be three or four days before taking
> another dose! Take it every two or three hours, the small quantities,
> for two or three days, then leave it off altogether for two or three days!
>
> 644-1

Small amounts, taken often, are more effective than one large dose
taken at once. What is a possible explanation for this advice?

> . . . Not sufficient that this becomes rancid in the system, see, but that
> acts as a lubricant and as a food for the digestive system . . .   257-13

As a laxative, it is to be taken no more or no less than what one's
body can assimilate. Belching or feeling nauseous indicates that too
much has been consumed; in that case, reduce the amount. Usually the
individual was told to continue the small doses " . . . until there is good
evacuation from the alimentary canal . . . " (5146–1)

Numerous other references in the readings mention the use of olive
oil as a food for its quality to easily assimilate and its helpfulness " . . . to
any intestinal disturbance . . . " (567–7) As a cathartic (a medicine to
stimulate or increase the frequency of bowel evacuation—a purgative
or laxative), it is considered the least irritating and most effective remedy in improving one's eliminations, as noted in this reading:

> ... For, as we have oft indicated, the Olive Oil is a real food value for the whole of the digestive system, as well as an assistant to the better eliminations or activities of the peristaltic movement of the bowels themselves ...   538-69

The peristaltic movement refers to the wavelike motions alternating between muscular contraction and relaxation, by which the food content is moved throughout the alimentary canal. Olive oil, taken periodically in small quantities, assists this process and is good "medicine" for improving eliminations.

Anyone doing a series of **castor oil packs** is usually advised to ingest a one-time dose (or more) of olive oil after the final pack of the series is completed. Only a few readings mention taking it on the same days as the packs. (See also *Amount of Dosage of Olive Oil* in the chapter on "Castor Oil Pack.")

The purpose of taking the olive oil is " ... to purify or to drain the colon, as well as the gall duct ... " (852-18) Other readings note that it will " ... *cleanse* the alimentary canal ... " (704-1), " ... make for the coordinating of that produced by the absorption of the Castor Oil." (1034-1), and " ... eliminate the poisons and accumulations." (3527-1)

Though amounts of the oil varied, as mentioned earlier, the portion consumed is generally one that can be comfortably absorbed. Those with a history of gallbladder or liver trouble, according to Dr. Harold Reilly, are advised to ingest the minimum amount.

The most common suggestion for external applications of olive oil is as a lubricant for **massage**. (For more information and explanation *see* the chapter on "Massage.") One reading states succinctly:

> ... As given, as known and held by the ancients more than the present modes of medication, olive oil—properly prepared (hence pure olive oil should always be used)—is one of the most effective agents for stimulating muscular activity, or mucus-membrane activity, that may be applied to a body ...   440-3

Another reading adds: " ... for few oils there be that are as much food for the tissue and muscular forces of the body as of the olive oil . . . " (5498–3)

Considered a "skin food" (noted in several readings), olive oil can also be combined with other substances (such as tincture of myrrh, castor oil, wintergreen oil, or peanut oil) and rubbed into the body, as much as the body can absorb. Its absorption makes for greater elasticity, prevents adhesions from forming, relieves soreness, stimulates blood and lymph circulation, and is " . . . very strengthening to the body . . . " (839–1) (*See also* the chapters "Peanut Oil Massage," "Myrrh," and "Castor Oil Pack.")

The **apple diet** consists of eating only raw apples and drinking lots of water for three days. (*See* the chapter "Apple Diet" for further information.) On the last day of this diet, that evening at bedtime, one is to drink a " . . . big dose of Olive Oil." (1409–9) or " . . . half a cup (teacup) of Pure Olive Oil." (1622–1) According to the readings, the olive oil will help to cleanse all toxicity from the system.

DIRECTIONS FROM THE READINGS

For a sixty–five–year–old woman with arthritis, impaired circulation, poor eliminations, and spinal subluxations (reading given on January 20, 1934):

> First we would begin to take internally very small quantities *often* of pure olive oil, a few drops every hour during the waking state—not in the evenings, you see. Do this for a week to ten days, first. This is to add to the system those properties that will make for reactions through the whole of the alimentary canal and, specifically, to the glands or ducts where assimilation takes place; stimulating secretions in the area of the pancrean and the liver activity.   492-1

For an adult woman with uterine fibroid tumors, cystitis, and constipation (reading given on April 21, 1936):

> . . . Also we would massage across the abdomen, even from the stomach to the lower portion of the descending colon, with Olive Oil. Let the

body absorb same. This will not only aid in these directions but make for greater elasticity in the abdominal walls and make for the prevention of any adherence through the bodily system itself. Massage just what the body will absorb. At some periods it will be found that as much as a whole tablespoonful or two will be absorbed by the body, and at other periods only a very small quantity will be absorbed.   1140-2

For a sixty-six-year-old woman suffering from general debilitation and neuritis tendencies (reading given on December 22, 1943):

It would be well for this body . . . to have a three-day apple diet, even in its weakened condition we need to clear the system. For this will get rid of the tendencies for neuritic conditions in the joints of the body. Also take the Olive Oil after the three-day diet. But don't go without the apples—eat them—all you can—at least five or six apples each day, chew them up, scrape them well. Drink plenty of water, and follow the three-day diet with the big dose of Olive Oil.   1409-9

For a fifty-nine-year-old woman with stomach lacerations, poor eliminations, and spinal subluxations (reading given on September 24, 1932):

Then we would begin, when there is the reduction of the periods of Castor Oil packs, with small quantities of olive oil, that there may be the feeding of the intestinal system to produce proper peristaltic movement through the system. Take a teaspoonful three or four times each day.   1736-4

For a fifty-one-year-old registered nurse suffering from arthritis, cholecystitis, and toxemia (reading given on July 21, 1939):

On the fifth day—that is, after the Packs have been used for four days, you see—we would take two tablespoonsful of Olive Oil, to *eliminate* those conditions which will have arisen by the absorbing of the Castor Oil through the system. This does not mean that other eliminants should not be taken before then, if necessary, but take the two table-spoonsful of Olive Oil on the fifth day (not before), for this should follow the Packs, you see.   1953-1

TESTIMONIALS/RESULTS

Recipients of readings noted their struggles with using olive oil—from obtaining the real product with regard to its purity to feeling sick and nauseous when ingesting it. A number of them questioned Cayce for a reevaluation. Usually the instructions included limiting the amount—often because too much had been taken; smaller doses consumed every few hours would be better than one large dose. Here are several accounts of their reports:

Mrs. [1010], a sixty-five-year-old woman from Alabama, wrote to Edgar Cayce on September 12, 1936, to describe her experiences in following her reading of August 17, 1936:

" . . . I began the {castor} oil-packs treatment on Aug. 18 . . . after taking olive oil for three days {I} passed about a tablespoon of gall stones. All but a few were only the size of grape seeds, a few {were} the size of the tip of the little finger. They passed for three days. {On the} third day just a little sand or gravel. Never stopped work, only for two days. Am feeling quite well again . . .

"Have some pain in gall bladder and liver at times but not to amount to anything. As you say, the age of body and disease can never be completely cured, but those awful spells are gone for the present . . . "
1010-10, Report #2

An A.R.E. member, Ouida Smith, wrote this report on March 19, 1973:

"I was not taking any medication for arthritis, even though I have had this disease for over 10 years.

"I recently started drinking olive oil. I took approximately 6 tablespoons a day (during the day) for 2 weeks, then I took 1 tablespoon a day for 2 weeks. The pain in every joint was gone. I stopped this procedure, feeling that maybe the arthritis may have been arrested as some cases do.

"After 3 weeks the pain started to return. I knew it must be the olive oil, so I started taking 3 tablespoons a day for 1 week, then discontinued dosage. After 2 weeks the pain was only slight but returning. I took only 3 tablespoons just one day a week. All I take now is 3 tablespoons for 1 day and it lasts 1 week and no pain for this period.

"I sincerely hope this will aid in finding help for people who suffer from this disease."   951-2, Report #22

Mr. [5642], thirty–one years old, in March of 1927 responded to a questionnaire as a follow–up to his reading, which he received on December 31, 1926:

" . . . I followed your directions . . . to the extent of using spinal massages of Olive Oil and Myrrh, which were prescribed with very satisfactory results and intend to continue using same. One of my most important nerves of {*my*} nervous system {*oftentimes*} does not function as it should, causing temporary fainting spells or a form of epilepsy caused from shell shock or fractured skull . . . I am obtaining surprising results from spinal massage . . . My case is epilepsy, not the hereditary kind but caused from my fractured skull . . . "

5642-1, Report #4

ADDITIONAL INFORMATION

A prime component of the Mediterranean Diet, olive oil is a natural juice and the only vegetable oil that can be consumed as is, freshly pressed from the fruit. The olive tree, which has been cultivated for centuries for its oil–bearing fruit, is a small evergreen native to the Mediterranean area (except for Egypt). It has lance–shaped leaves and is mentioned a number of times in the Bible; an olive branch is considered a symbol of peace. As seen in the previous information, the oil can be applied both internally and externally.

Mayo Clinic dietitian, Katherine Zeratsky, RD, LD, writes:

"All types of olive oil provide monounsaturated fat, but 'extra-virgin' or 'virgin' olive oils are the least processed forms. As a result, they contain the highest levels of polyphenols, a powerful antioxidant . . .

"According to the Food and Drug Administration (FDA), consuming about 2 tablespoons (23 grams) of olive oil a day may reduce your risk of heart disease. You can get the most benefit by substituting olive oil for saturated fats rather than just adding more olive oil to your diet." ("Ask a Food and Nutrition Specialist," MayoClinic.com)

OTHER USES FOR OLIVE OIL

The olive oil seasoning on a **salad** " . . . is a food, and not a fat . . . " (460-4) and gives " . . . proper toning of the digestive system . . . " (2092-1) As noted in the *Amount of Dosage* section, the readings recommend one teaspoon to be added to the salad.

An olive oil **hair tonic** or any olive oil-based **shampoo**, according to the readings, is preferable to other products on the market. For an itchy scalp, one woman was advised to rub into her scalp some olive oil placed on the tips of her fingers (514-2). One sixty-year-old woman, who received a reading in 1931 regarding her own hair tonic preparation, asked about the use of olive oil and was offered this suggestion:

> . . . Do not have too much of the olive oil, or too much of the coconut oil, or too much of *any* of the oils—but sufficient that they give their *lustre* in their proper relationships.   658-6

Other readings' extracts offer this information:

> (Q) What shampoo should be used for hair?
> (A) Any that carries sufficient of the olive oils . . .   275-27

> (Q) How can I best care for my hair and keep it light, and from turning dark at the roots?
> (A) Use an Olive Oil Shampoo. This as we find would be the better way. Shampoo it at least once each week.   1431-2

Enemas administered with an olive oil base, for one individual, would relieve pressure and irritation from the kidneys and bladder (505-1). Another was advised to have a gentle enema, placing olive oil (about half a pint) in the first enema " . . . so that there may be the relaxing." (1523-9) One reading states:

> We would also give *enemas* of olive oil to relieve the distress as is seen in the muscular forces in the descending colon.   340-7

For a forty-year-old man, suffering from toxemia and past physical problems, the reading, 3484-1, advised a **cabinet sweat bath** in which a little olive oil mixed with witch hazel was added to the boiling water to create a fume for a moist heat bath. Creating this kind of moist heat is one of the few times in the readings when olive oil is used in such a way.

Four instances of using **flannel cloth packs** that were saturated in hot olive oil were mentioned. For one seventy-year-old woman, suffering from colitis, the cloth was to be placed " . . . on abdomen and side . . . " to " . . . assist more in breaking up these attacks and give more stimulation to the walls of the intestinal tract, by increasing the circulation." (3776-10) In an earlier reading, she was told to place the pack " . . . across the intestine and lower bowel, where these troubles show in the walls of intestine . . . " (3776-9)

A two-year-old girl, also suffering from colitis along with fever, received her fifth reading on June 3, 1928. It noted that whenever she had pain or " . . . a hardening of the region about this portion where trouble occurs; that is, in the right side, in the ascending colon . . . ," she was to " . . . apply hot packs, or very warm packs, just so it will not burn the body . . . " (608-5) The mother later reported that her daughter was much improved.

Another woman was told to mix equal amounts of olive and peanut oil and apply the heated " . . . heavy flannel or toweling . . . " pack to areas on her back that needed relaxation; she was advised to do this each time prior to her osteopathic adjustments. (2825-1)

In the last case, drops of spirits of camphor were added to the heated oil, and the pack placed " . . . across the lower end of stomach, liver, and the right side . . . ," changing the pack every twenty to twenty-five min-utes, until a reaction was produced in the liver. (4611-1) This case was for an eight-year-old girl suffering with fever and cold, whose parents obtained this emergency physical reading; coincidentally it was ob-tained on June 11, just eight days after [608]'s reading mentioned previ-ously. Three days later her mother reported that [4611] was " . . . getting along very nicely now." (4611-1, Report #1)

Although the adjective "pure" to describe the type of olive oil was mentioned a little over one hundred times in the readings and "virgin" was mentioned just once, it can be assumed that the readings meant for the olive oil to be of high quality, the least refined, and the least pro-cessed.

Onion Juice

Concentrated juices derived from certain vegetables, fruits, and meats can be utilized as a form of medicine for the body. Noted in the readings are the juices from beef, grapes, liver, potato peelings, as well as onions. This concoction is not to be confused with broth or soup, which can also be made from some of these food sources, but is a definite juice that is extracted by boiling the substance, either in Patapar paper or by steaming it. As with other concentrated juices, only small amounts are taken at one time.

A further note on the cooking process: In some readings, Cayce stressed that the onions should not be placed directly into boiling water; this was probably to preserve the juices and keep the extract in a concentrated form—hence, the recommendation to use Patapar paper.

Nearly twenty individuals were advised to take onion juice as part of their health regimen.

INDICATIONS

Adenoiditis, bronchitis, catarrh, circulation incoordination, cold, congestion, debilitation, pneumonia, throat problems, tonsillitis, tuberculosis, whooping cough

MATERIALS NEEDED

Large white onion or several onions (up to six); fresh, if possible
Pot or container—to steam or boil the onions
Small container—to collect and store the juice
Patapar paper (optional)—parchment paper in which to place the
onions for boiling

FREQUENCY OF DOSAGE

Every 30 minutes; every few hours; every 20 minutes to ½ hour;
every 1 to 2 hours; every 1½ to 2 hours; every 4 hours; 1, 2, or 3 times a
day; just before retiring

AMOUNT OF DOSAGE

Small quantities; a few drops; 2, 3, 4, or 5 drops; 3 to 4 sips every 2 or
3 hours; 20 drops; ¼ to ½ teaspoon; 1 or 2 teaspoons; 1 tablespoon

LENGTH OF TIME OF APPLICATION

Take 2 or 3 times each day for 3 or 4 days; take for 3 or 4 days once a
day for 1 week; once a day for 1 week, off 1 week, then repeat

EXPECTED EFFECTS/PURPOSES

Relaxes the body (for sleep)
Removes inflammation
Clarifies the blood
Acts upon the digestive system
Cleanses and clarifies the respiratory system
Relieves heaviness in the chest, throat, and nasal passages
Clears throat and mucous membranes
Stimulates the nervous system
Promotes better eliminations
Strengthens the body

DIRECTIONS

Boil or steam one or several onions—fresh, if possible, or of the Spanish variety. The onion or onions may be placed in Patapar paper, tied

with a bowknot, set in water, and boiled lightly. The juice is then squeezed or pressed out of the onion after the boiling or steaming. Collect the juice in a small container and sip small amounts throughout the day (see *Frequency of Dosage* and *Amount of Dosage*). Some readings mention adding a little lemon juice, sugar, or other sweetener like honey or saccharin to the onion juice. Keep the juice in a cool place and make it fresh daily.

DIRECTIONS FROM THE READINGS

For a seventy-one-year-old woman suffering from bronchial pneumonia and debilitation (reading given on September 9, 1937):

> Then we would boil onions in Patapar Paper and give the syrup of same as an internal effect upon the digestive system. The large white onion for such usage, pressed to obtain the juice from same. The sips of the onion juice would be given about an hour and a half to two hours apart; about a quarter to half a teaspoonful. This will act upon the digestive forces of the body.   326-10

For a sixty-three-year-old male aggravated by congestion and a cold (reading given on November 28, 1929):

> Well, too, were onion juice given to clarify the throat. Boil onions and press the juice from same, sweetening same just a tiny bit. Teaspoonful at the time will clear the throat and the {*mucous*} membranes in the bronchia . . .   2504-5

For a sixty-three-year-old male with bronchitis tendencies and circulatory problems (reading given on May 13, 1936):

> We would begin with the use of onion juices; juices squeezed from boiled onions—or onions boiled in Patapar Paper. And eat the onions as well as drink the juice from same. Let this be a part of one meal each day for a week, leave off for a week and then take again; the onions cooked in that way and manner, you see, to preserve their juices. Fresh

onions if possible; if not, those that are well preserved—or the Spanish variety. These properties will act upon the circulation and the
whole of the pulmonary reaction, as to produce a better elimination.

909-2

TESTIMONIALS/RESULTS

No supplemental material exists in the readings regarding specifically the taking of onion juice. There are only a few references to following directions in the readings, which included a recommendation
for onion juice; for example:

In reply to a questionnaire sent out by Gladys Davis, a wife on September 16, 1940, wrote about her husband's experience (he was suffering from tuberculosis):

> " . . . Every time he had a reading it was perfect in its analysis of Mr.
> [572]'s condition. We followed the first few readings and he got great
> help. I believe he would have been living today if we had faithfully car-
> ried out the readings instead of putting him again into the hands of
> the doctors."   572-9, Report #2

A woman, also in response to a questionnaire and who was suffering
from bronchial pneumonia, noted on May 26, 1938:

> " . . . I followed the suggestions in the reading for four or five years. I
> am now very much better."   326-9, Report #6

ADDITIONAL INFORMATION

Notations made at the end of several readings indicate that onions
contain sulfur, iodine, iron, and calcium. In combination with other
vegetables they are designated as "body building" and help to control
acid buildup in the body.

Often in the readings one discovers hidden treasures—comments
made almost casually, yet bringing more of a focus and greater attention to a particular subject. These treasures are "hidden" because usually they are not indexed in such a way to draw one's attention to them;

indeed, they are observed by the reader who almost inadvertently happens upon them.

Such is the case with a question–and–answer exchange in reading 5671-16 (see the Appendix under the heading "Whooping Cough/Pneumonia" for the complete answer). The recipient of the reading, a thirty-four-year-old woman, asked what she could give her baby for whooping cough. After mentioning some drops to be taken orally and a massage oil to be applied externally, the answer concludes:

> . . . When the nausea comes, if there is given the juice of onions—not with that that is boiled in water, but heated and the juice pressed out—this is the best thing for pneumonia that may be given!   5671-16

Unfortunately in her three follow-up readings no more mention is made of the baby—its sex, age, or any results with the treatments recommended. Yet a strong endorsement is made about the beneficial effects of onion juice as a remedy for pneumonia.

See also the chapter on "Onion Poultice" for further information on onions.

Onion Poultice

A poultice is a soft, hot, moist mass of some substance (like an onion) that is spread on a cloth and applied to an area of the body. It is designed to hold prolonged, moist warmth between two cloth layers. The presence of heat aids the absorption of medicinal substances by the skin.

The bulbous onion, along with its numerous relatives (garlic, leeks, chives, etc.), belongs to the lily family. All of its edible forms, used as a food since ancient times, have distinctive flavors and odors. When a warm onion poultice is placed on the chest, the vapors and heat improve breathing by clearing congested airways—one of the most irritating symptoms of a bad cold. Onions also contain large amounts of sulfur compounds, making them good detoxifiers and antibiotics. Despite the adverse influence onions may have on one's social life, its positive effects on health far outweigh the negative!

For twenty-six individuals, onion poultices were a suggested therapy.

INDICATIONS
Asthma, bronchitis, cold/congestion, fever, flu (aftereffects), frac-

tured ribs, injury (from a fall), lung adhesions, measles, pleurisy, pneumonia, tonsillitis, toxemia, tuberculosis

MATERIALS NEEDED

Onions—large, raw, chopped rather fine; old rather than new; enough to cover desired area

Two cloths—gauze, linen, course cotton, or cheesecloth—one on top of the onion slices and one on the bottom; or one large piece of cloth to be folded over the entire onion mass

Yellow corn meal (preferred)—or white corn meal or yellow oat meal (½ teaspoon up to 1 tablespoon)

Patapar paper (optional)—parchment paper in which to place the onions for boiling

Large plate or tray (optional)—to transport poultice from stove to chest

Heating pad (optional)—to maintain heat

FREQUENCY OF APPLICATION

Once daily up to three times daily (multiple applications require freshly made poultices); leave on until condition improves, inflammation subsides, or phlegm is cleared; remove, bathe off, or wash area (probably with tepid water), then reapply with fresh poultice, if necessary

LENGTH OF TIME OF APPLICATION

Ten minutes, 30 minutes, 1 hour for two days, 1½ to 2 hours, 2 to 3 hours, 4 to 5 hours, until improvements noted

LOCATION OF APPLICATION

Front and/or back of lungs, lobes of lung, trachea and bronchial areas; kidneys and lumbar area; across the chest, but not over the breast; throat; right side of abdomen: liver/gall bladder/cecum area; injured, painful area (from a fall)

SIZE OF PACK

One-fourth of an inch to one-half of an inch thick, appropriate size to cover area

EXPECTED EFFECTS/PURPOSES

Eases breathing
Breaks up lung congestion
Draws, disseminates, and dissipates fluid
Stimulates circulation
Reduces feeling of fullness or heaviness in chest
Helps reduce shortness of breath
Dissipates accumulations
Relieves pressure in ear

DIRECTIONS

Chop up raw onions (rather fine), using enough pieces of the onion to cover desired area one-fourth to one-half inch thick. Heat the onions slightly in a pot without water or place them in Patapar paper. If using the latter, tie the ends of the paper together with a string, making a bowtie at the top. Set the Patapar package in water and heat it—not cooking it but gently sautéing it—so that it becomes juicy. Have some cloth or gauze laid out on a large tray or plate ready to receive the onion mass. Remove the onions from the heat.

Sprinkle in corn meal—yellow is preferred (one reading recommended white). Add enough of the meal to hold the onion mix together, from one-half teaspoon up to one tablespoon. Then pour and spread the onion mass onto the cloth, folding the edges to hem it in and secure the mixture. If necessary, place another cloth on top and fold the edges of both cloths together to contain the mass. Place the warm poultice directly against the skin, and leave it on for the determined amount of time. Add a heating pad on top of the poultice, if desired. Wash the area afterward with tepid water. If the condition persists, reapply later with a fresh poultice.

DIRECTIONS FROM THE READINGS

For a sixty-two-year-old male suffering the aftereffects of flu (reading given on May 2, 1943):

About an hour at the time, each day for about two days, we would apply the Onion Poultices over the liver, the gall duct, and extending to the caecum area; prepared in this manner:

Prepare a thin gauze or cloth of sufficient size to cover this area. Cut up onions very fine; heat them, not cook them too much but heat them; mixing with them—for this quantity—about a tablespoonful of corn meal—preferably the yellow corn meal. Spread this on the cloth, covering with a heavier cloth—warm, not too hot—and apply to the body.

After this has been on for some ten minutes (not in the beginning) apply an electric pad, and let this heat for at least thirty minutes more, see?

Then this may be cleansed off.   1561-22

For a forty-four-year-old male suffering with a cold and chest congestion (reading given on June 2, 1943):

Should there arise the filling, or the fullness in the chest, shortness of breath, apply an onion poultice over the area—to draw or to disseminate and dissipate the fluid. Chop onions rather fine, preferably using old onions rather than new ones. Then heat them; not too much, as to burn, but keep the oils in same. Sprinkle just a little yellow oat or corn meal in same, so as to make a poultice of the onions—having a layer of onions half an inch thick on plain gauze. Apply this for an hour at the time.

If this persists, keep on adding more of these poultices, for it will dissipate the accumulations.   3021-2

For a fifty-six-year-old woman suffering from pneumonia (reading given on April 2, 1943):

On the frontal portion we would put an Onion Poultice, for activity to the circulation through the breast, the chest and the lungs, see? Use large onions chopped rather fine, and heated—not cooked, but heated so as to get the juice out of same though leave the juice in the poultice, see. Mix with a little yellow corn meal, about a tablespoonful—this prepared on gauze that would extend from the throat down to the end of the breast bone, and spread across the chest—not over the breast but across the chest, around the breast, see? In four to five hours change this, make another fresh Onion Poultice and apply. There should not be required more than the one change, but do put on a fresh poultice in about four to five hours.   303-40

For a two-month-old male infant with a bad cough and cold (reading given on March 17, 1940):

Almost immediately, or as soon as practical, apply an Onion Poultice over the chest, as well as between the shoulders. Do not make the poultice too strong, else it would be too severe for the developing body. Chop the onions very fine, heat them—or cook them until they are about half done, you see; keeping most of the juice with same—preferably cook them in Patapar Paper, this would be the better way. Then mix just sufficient raw corn meal with same to make into a poultice, not too thick but just sufficient to allow the poultice to be applied—between gauze—directly to the body. For this body, preferably use the *yellow* corn meal. Apply the poultice while it is still warm, you see. Leave it on for at least thirty minutes. Then if there is not a change in the congestion, in twenty-four hours, put it on again—making a fresh poultice, of course.   2148-1

TESTIMONIALS/RESULTS

From "How the Readings Helped My Life"—emailed to A.R.E. on March 3, 2006:

"My daughter suffers from chronic asthma, to the point of nearly dying five years ago. She is thirty years old, and when she begins to get a cold, the first place it settles is in her chest. There seems to be no stopping its progression there, even with her inhaler and other asthma medications. So we always hold our breath when she starts this downward spiral into her asthma attack. Last month when she told me she was feeling her chest tighten up, I relayed to her what I had just read .

.. about onion poultices being helpful for breaking up chest congestion. Her husband made the poultice for her, and she wore it on her
chest twice during a weekend. Her chest became beet red and warm,
and she said it broke up her congestion that first day. She never went
into her usual pattern of tightness ending in asthma. She was so grateful for this little-known remedy, and said her apartment smelled like
an Italian kitchen—an added bonus!"

Jenny Moe, San Rafael, California

A follow-up reading for Mrs. [303], three and a half months later (*see*
information from reading 303-40 above), indicated that the lung congestion had not been entirely eliminated, " . . . but there are no active
forces there. The circulation is much improved." (303-41)

ADDITIONAL INFORMATION

In a reading for his twelve-year-old daughter, one father asked if
either onion or mustard packs would dissolve the fluid in her chest. The
reading stated:

. . . While the mustard makes for more of a superficial stimulation, the
onion would be penetrating and not as irritating . . .   632-13

OTHER USES FOR ONIONS

As part of one's diet, onions—both raw and cooked—are recommended in the Cayce readings. Generally, raw onions are eaten, along
with other raw vegetables, at the noon meal, and cooked onions are to
be consumed at the evening meal. Even the juice of the onion can be
drunk (*see* the chapter on "Onion Juice"), mostly to allay respiratory and
digestive imbalances. In addition to their sulfur content, mentioned earlier, onions also contain iodine, iron, and calcium.

Not only do they help prevent a buildup of acidity in the body when
combined with other vegetables, they are also "body building" (815-1)
and "carry roughage" (719-2), thus assisting better eliminations and purifying the system. Along with carrots, green peas, green beans, and
beets, onions " . . . have a direct bearing upon the optic forces." (3552-1),

helping to improve one's eyesight and general vision.

Onions can also eradicate small pinworms from the system. " . . . They'll scare 'em away!" reading (308-2) states.

One woman asked, "Since onions are supposed to be good for your blood and otherwise, why do they cause such ill smelling gases?" Cayce's answer was: "From the most foul at times comes the most beautiful lilies." (457-9)

Peanut Oil Massage

As a lubricant for massage, peanut oil is the one substance most often recommended in the Cayce health information—either by itself or in combination with other oils. The adjective *lowly* was used several times in the readings to describe it, yet peanut oil has quite a variety of accomplishments despite earning that designation. Usually recommended for the prevention of arthritis and rheumatism, it is also helpful for paralysis, dermatitis, and the supplying of energies to the body. Several readings also note that, unlike other oils, peanut oil " . . . does not become rancid . . . " on the skin. (2642-1)

It is mentioned in over six hundred readings, primarily suggested as a massage oil, but in a few instances it was recommended to be ingested orally as an eliminant, internally for enemas, or used as a cooking oil for fish and fowl.

INDICATIONS
Apoplexy, arthritis, blemishes or bumps on skin, burns, cholecystitis, coronary occlusion, dermatitis, dry skin, epilepsy, fatigue, general debilitation, glandular disturbances, heart condition, impaired locomotion, incoordination of nervous system, low vitality, meno-

pause, multiple sclerosis, neuritis, numbness in legs, palsy, paralysis, Parkinson's disease, polio, poor circulation, poor eliminations, rash, rheumatism, ringing in head and ears, sore and tight muscles, stiff joints, stomach ulcer, stress, stroke, swelling (feet), toxemia, varicose veins, weakness in knees and legs

CONTRAINDICATIONS

One of the most common food allergens and may cause severe reactions in sensitive people, avoid peanut oil massage on same day as osteopathic adjustments, avoid using it for a massage during the same period when taking it as an enema, see also *Contraindications* in the chapter "Massage"

MATERIALS NEEDED

Referral to or recommendation of a professional massage therapist
Bottle of pure peanut oil
Massage table or folding table draped with sheets and towels
Bowl, saucer, or cup—to put oil in
Grain alcohol—for a rubdown after the massage (optional)
Hand towel—to rub the back following alcohol application (optional)

FREQUENCY OF APPLICATION

Twice a day; each morning and each evening; each afternoon; daily; every other day; 1, 2, or 3 times a week; occasionally; every 10 days for 2, 3, or 4 months

AMOUNT OF DOSAGE

What the skin and body can absorb, 2 tablespoons

WHEN TO TAKE THE PEANUT OIL MASSAGE

After a foot bath, an Epsom salt pack, or a thorough workout; after an ultraviolet light and green glass treatment (peanut oil and witch hazel); after hot and cold packs, lying in a warm bath, taking a tepid bath, or taking a walk (exercise); each day when taking Atomidine; following a cabinet steam/fume bath; following a series of osteopathic adjustments or use of the Wet–Cell Appliance; just before retiring; on days when castor oil packs are not given; 4 or 5 days before menstrual period (massage limbs); " . . . after any service in water, massage the hands with the lowly peanut oil . . . " (1309-6)

LENGTH OF TIME OF APPLICATION

Twenty to 30 minutes; ½ hour to 1½ hours; 30 to 40 minutes; regularly for 6 months, then off for 2 to 3 months; once a week for 10 to 15 weeks

LOCATION OF APPLICATION

Abdomen; across all the areas of the spine; across the clavicle, the hips, the sacral area, the stomach; along the cerebrospinal system; along the sympathetic system rather than the cerebrospinal system; diaphragm; feet, ankles, heels, instep, and toes; from frontal area to pit of stomach; hips, elbows, hands; joints, neck, the ribs; limbs; lower back; temples, face, shoulders, along the spine, and arms; sciatic center to below the knees; under the knees; where the hot and cold packs were applied

EXPECTED EFFECTS/PURPOSES

Makes the skin, muscles, nerves, and tendons more pliable

Aids in stimulating better eliminations

Strengthens " . . . the activities of the structural body itself." (2968-1)

Supplies " . . . a food for the nerves *and* muscular forces . . . " (2321-2)

Gives strength, vitality, and energy to the body as well as rest

Provides " . . . nutriment, elasticity and activity to the cerebrospinal system." (2642-1)

Helps to revive "the glandular forces" (2529-1)

Replenishes depleted nerve energies

Balances the mental and spiritual aspects of the body

Aids " . . . in better appetite, better growth, and better activities throughout the body." (1788-9)

Stimulates muscles and tendons at the ends and in the joints of bones

Allays " . . . the irritation produced by the fume bath . . . " (2421-1)

Coordinates " . . . the nerve and the muscular forces of the body . . . " (318-7)

Assists the body system to rebuild and replenish

DIRECTIONS

As stated in the chapter on "Massage," due to individual differences in one's health condition, age, sex, and severity of symptoms, it would be impossible to describe a massage that fits everyone. The suggestion is made, therefore, to follow the directions in chapter 9 of Dr. Harold Reilly's book *The Edgar Cayce Handbook for Health* as a place to begin. Examining several Cayce readings referring to a specific ailment as well as taking into account their descriptions of what areas to focus on during the massage is also beneficial. For further information on the Cayce/Reilly® approach to massage, read the *Directions* section in the chapter on "Massage."

A few more notations on massage are added here. Occasionally the readings suggest an alcohol rub at the end of the massage to help close the pores. This alcohol is not your usual isopropyl rubbing alcohol but is grain alcohol, as some readings clarify. One way of administering this rubdown is to have a hand towel handy, pour a small portion of the grain alcohol into your palms, quickly rub your palms together to spread the alcohol onto your fingers, then briskly and swiftly in circular movements spread it over the client's back. (The client will be lying face down.) The alcohol, of course, evaporates quickly, so just a few circles will be needed. Grab the towel in a wad and quickly cover the back area in short and vigorous back-and-forth motions. It will be stimulating and cooling, increasing alertness as well as removing excess oil from the back. Afterward, cover the back with a sheet.

As with other therapies, the massage should be " . . . lovingly, carefully administered . . . " (2642-1), done " . . . not hurriedly, not as something to be gotten through with . . . " (1789-8), but prayerfully, and with gentleness, for " . . . just a gentle massage . . . will rest the body much." (1505-4) Of course, in following any particular regimen, the advice is usually to be consistent and persistent, as well as thorough. The practitioner, then, is to maintain these attitudes and " . . . give suggestions that

are constructive, creative, as of body, mind *and* spiritual awakening . . . "
(1990–6)

DIRECTIONS FROM THE READINGS

For a forty-year-old male with tuberculosis, impaired locomotion, and general debilitation (reading given on December 5, 1940):

> Across the hips, and down the limbs and feet, we would use a massage with Peanut Oil; not a combination of oils, but just the Peanut Oil. This as a food for the nerves *and* muscular forces will be most beneficial.
>
> Begin with the body lying prone upon face. Begin at about the 2nd and 3rd lumbar, and very thoroughly—in a circular motion—massage all that the body will absorb—across the sacral and the rump itself, and into those areas about where the pelvic bone joins with the lower limbs. Give this deep, thorough massage each day. Not that much oil is put on at a time—just what may be adhering to the fingers by dipping them in same, in a shallow container—as a saucer or the like. Continue this along the sciatic nerves to that portion under the knee; then along the muscular forces in the calf of the leg, coming down on either side; massaging away from the body rather than toward the body, but in a circular motion all the while. Extend the massage below the calf of the leg upon either side of the small bone and tendon to the heel, and then about the ankle, into that portion of the foot and heel—the instep portion; and then upon the back, over the limbs, in the same way and manner, especially with the knee, the ankle, and the upper portion of the foot and the front bursa, or in the foot, or that under the great toe and across the foot there.
>
> This massage we would give *thoroughly* each day. Take thirty minutes or more to give this treatment. For this body, it would be preferable to give this each afternoon, for it would rest the body better and he would feel better—at least after the third or fourth treatment. 2321-2

For an adult male who was a patient in a sanitarium, suffering from nervous system incoordination (reading given on November 5, 1940):

Each evening, for twenty to thirty minutes, give a spinal rub. This would be given—by the nurse—when the body is prepared for sleeping, or for bed. Rub with pure Peanut Oil, in a circular motion, down either side of the spine. This will not only aid in the absorption of this to create a better superficial circulation, but will aid in making better coordinations between the reflexes of the sympathetic system *and* the cerebrospinal system.   2387-2

For a fifty-five-year-old woman with malaria and poor assimilations (reading given on October 22, 1941):

(Q) Is Peanut Oil good for me to take internally?
(A) Let's rub it on at present. It will be very well to use it in the enemas, if so desired. This is a helpful influence internally and externally, but let's not mix it while we are rubbing it on. Let's absorb this, unless—as indicated—there is the desire to use in the enemas that will cleanse the colon occasionally, which would be good for the body.   303-26

For a forty-year-old male suffering from poor assimilations (reading given on December 29, 1941):

Also have fish and fowl, but these prepared with the reinforced vitamins in the flour, the meal or the like. Use not the vegetable oils in the cooking, but either the peanut oil or the Parkay margarine—for this especially carries D in a manner that conforms with these properties in preparation for assimilation by the body.   826-14

TESTIMONIALS/RESULTS

Reports in the Cayce files corroborate many of the statements made in the readings. From Mrs. Mary Sutter comes a letter dated April 22, 1977, in which she writes:

" . . . I had (such) a bad case of arthritis in my right hip and leg that I was living on pain pills. I tried peanut oil. I used the oil Friday—Sunday, Tuesday . . . Wednesday. I got up in the morning, and I couldn't

believe the pain was completely gone. That was over a year ago and I
have had none since . . . "   5361-1, Report #5

Another letter, dated December 9, 1971, was written by William F.
Keller, who described his experience with peanut oil:

"As a rheumatoid arthritic I have found (pure peanut oil) to be of great
benefit to my condition. After using (it) as a massaging oil for several
years, I have to agree with Cayce's belief that it not only lubricates, but
heals as well. I am sure that had I known about the oil in this use, I
would have been spared much misery.
    " . . . Why isn't the use of pure peanut oil to reduce joint inflamma-
tion and pain in arthritis better known? Does the medical profession
spurn it as a home remedy? . . . "   3363-1, Report #2

The following account is a verbal report on January 3, 1947, from Mr.
[1467], who was thirty–six years old when he received his eleventh reading on October 25, 1941. He explains his response to the advice given him:

"I had a scar from an appendix operation, which had healed, but sometimes when bending over . . . I would get a terrific cramp in my side.
This would form a knot . . . about the size of my fist, and the only way I
could get rid of it would be to massage it. After the reading suggested
peanut oil, I started massaging with it about two or three times a week.
In about a year the condition was completely cured. The cramps have
not bothered me since, and this was about six years ago."
                                                              1467-11, Report #4

ADDITIONAL INFORMATION

Though some people may think of them as nuts that grow on trees,
peanuts are actually legumes, like peas. The peanut plant produces self-
pollinating yellow flowers, which form "pegs" that eventually grow
stems and push into the ground. Nuts develop inside the brittle pods,
which contain one to three edible seeds. At harvest time, between September and October, the peanuts are dug out of the ground, dried in

the sun for two to three days, and then separated from the vines by a combine. Shellers clean and grade the raw nuts before they are sold on the market.

The nutlike seeds have a high protein content and are a source of vitamins D and B-complex, without undesirable cholesterol. Peanuts also contain six essential vitamins, seven essential minerals, and are an excellent source of resveratrol (also present in red wine).

Chemically classified as monounsaturated, the oil extracted from the nuts is suitable for a wide range of cooking temperatures and is less prone to deterioration than polyunsaturated oils.

The process of extraction affects the oil's nutritional content, storage life, and quality. Mechanical or expeller extraction is the preferred method. In this process an expeller press crushes the nuts, raising the temperature of the oil to 185° to 200°F (85° to 93.3°C); the heat makes the pressing more efficient. Other manufacturers may produce a "cold-pressed" oil, meaning that additional external heat was not utilized to extract the oil. In this process, cold water, run through the expeller, keeps the temperature of the oil from rising. There is no legal or binding definition of "cold pressed," and oils may be so labeled even when temperatures are quite high during pressing. The term "cold pressed" does not appear in the readings; several times, however, the oil to be used was referred to as *pure* peanut oil. Technically, *pure* means "unmixed, free from any adulterant, clear."

Caution must be observed, as peanuts are one of the most common food allergens and, as stated earlier, may cause severe reactions in sensitive people. According to the Web site eHow.com, however, oil that is contaminated with peanut protein may not be safe, but pure peanut oil is usually nonallergenic.

The most familiar Cayce excerpt is the often-quoted: "Those who would take a peanut oil rub {massage} each week need never fear arthritis." (1158-31) A similar reading calls peanut oil a "food" and with regular massages, " . . . there will never be—or need never be any fear of neuritic or arthritic tendencies—which, of course, are a natural tendency where there is any glandular disturbance." (2582-1) A third excerpt states that a peanut oil massage is " . . . beneficial to all, and . . . tends to be a preventative of rheumatic or arthritic tendencies . . . " (1309-7), probably because—as stated in a fourth reading—it is " . . . a stimul{us} to the muscular and tendon forces at the ends and in the joints of the bones . . . " (2956-1)

See *Testimonials/Results* which seem to corroborate these statements.

OTHER USES FOR PEANUT OIL

Though primarily used externally as a massage oil, peanut oil was also recommended in three cases to be taken internally as "an eliminant" (257-233), just a few drops ingested daily, combined or alternated with olive oil. One person (1788-5) was told that this combination would help assimilation and strengthen liver and kidney activity (*see* reading 1788-5 on the following page for complete quote). One reading suggested it as a cooking oil for fish and fowl (826-14), while another recommended its use " . . . in the enemas, if so desired . . . " (303-26)—but not during the period when one was using it for massages. Since peanut oil is mentioned in 612 readings, these few cases are exceptional and specialized instances of its use.

Reports also mention two physicians, and one " . . . recommended Planters Peanut Oil to all his burn patients . . . ," to be massaged in three times a day. (2015-10, Report #14) This information appeared in a letter dated June 28, 1974, from Dorothy Y. Bramble of Syracuse, N.Y., to Hugh Lynn Cayce. Another physician, according to a letter written by Edgar Cayce on January 16, 1939, offered peanut oil as part of his treatment for his multiple sclerosis patients. (849-33, Report #3)

As a side note, the Planters brand (from Suffolk, Virginia) was often suggested—not in the readings but in the follow-up information regarding suppliers—especially if the reading's recipient was having difficulty locating the oil. " . . . This is one of the best sources of supply that I know of . . . ," Cayce wrote to Mrs. [4009] on December 17, 1943. (4009-1, Background #4) Today most health food stores carry peanut oil.

The two most recommended oils in the readings, peanut and olive, were sometimes used together—for example, in equal amounts as a massage oil—and also alternated. Here are two extracts describing the comparison between them:

(Q) Is peanut oil taken internally as beneficial as olive oil?
(A) Peanut Oil is a lubricant and not a food as olive oil is. In some conditions it would be very well. As an eliminant it is very good. As a food value in some conditions it is more harmful than beneficial.

257-233

It will be well for this body to be given and to *retain,* as it were, a little Olive Oil each day; just a few drops will be most helpful for the body—as would be, alternated with same, the Peanut Oil. It is well that there be kept this activity so that there may be the better reaction with the whole of the hepatic circulation. One to two drops should be sufficient each day, see? One day give the Olive Oil, the next day the Peanut Oil, and so on. These act with the assimilating system and are strengthening to the activity of liver *and* kidneys, and thus will make for better conditions through the body.   1788-5

Other combinations made with peanut oil include grain alcohol, cod liver oil, and witch hazel, while certain formulas include a number of additional ingredients, such as sassafras oil, pine needle oil, tincture of benzoin, rosewater, liquefied lanolin, Russian White Oil, and other substances. These formulas are mentioned in individual readings for specific conditions.

Indeed, the lowly peanut oil has a worth beyond measure.

Potato Poultice

A poultice is a moist, soft mass (sometimes heated) of some substance—like a potato—that is usually spread on or between cloths and applied to an area of the body. In the case of the potato poultice, the substance is not heated, is relatively cool (at room temperature), and consists largely of scraped potato skin with a little pulp included. It is used specifically for the eyes. No cloth is placed between the potato pieces and the eye, for the mass is placed directly against the skin over the closed eyelids.

About sixty readings recommend potato poultices for the eyes.

According to Dr. William McGarey, enzymes released by the act of scraping the potato can enhance lymph flow and circulation in and around the eyes. This improved circulation provides for better elimination that will help remove any infections or inflamed material from the eyes.

The frequency and length of time for the poultice application would depend upon one's condition. Keep up the treatments until the condition is relieved.

INDICATIONS

Any eye and lid irritations, blepharitis (commonly called a "sty"), blindness, burning or tired eyes, cataracts, conjunctivitis (one type is known as "pinkeye"), eye and vision problems, eye inflammation or infection, eye lesions, granulated lids, myopia, poor eyesight, retinitis pigmentosa

MATERIALS NEEDED

One medium-sized potato: fully matured Irish potato (not green or new); common white potato or baking potato, also known as Idaho potato or russet potato; one that never has been frozen and has not begun to sprout; pesticide free—well scrubbed, rinsed thoroughly, and air-dried

Gauze or bandage—to place over eye poultice (for use overnight or while relaxing in a chair)

Shredding grater (use fine shred) or kitchen knife—to scrape the potato

Two small cups, bowls, or containers—to hold potato scrapings

Small paper cups—to hold cotton balls and antiseptic solution for cleansing the eye sockets afterward

Towel or piece of plastic (optional)—to place under the head

Antiseptic (alkaline) solution (weakened)—boric acid or Glyco-Thymoline—to bathe area after removal of potato scrapings

Wet washcloth or cotton balls soaked in water—to remove possible stickiness following alkaline solution

FREQUENCY OF APPLICATION

Daily, every 3 hours, every other day, once or twice a week

LENGTH OF TIME OF APPLICATION

Ten minutes, 15 to 30 minutes, 30 to 40 minutes, overnight; keep up treatments for 1 week up to 3 or 4 months until condition is relieved

LOCATION OF APPLICATION

Place potato scrapings over closed eyes; fill eye sockets completely with the moist, mushy scrapings; fasten it in place with gauze or a bandage, if needed

SIZE OF PACK

Enough scrapings to fill eye sockets (about 2 tablespoons total); cover about ½ inch thick

EXPECTED EFFECTS/PURPOSES

Clears up eye or eyelid infection, irritation, or inflammation
Draws impurities from eye tissue
Clarifies membranes around eyes
Strengthens central nerves leading to optic nerves
Relieves eyestrain
Removes drosses from the eyes

DIRECTIONS

Choose a medium-sized Irish potato (a white-skinned potato—also called baking, Idaho, or russet potato). Scrub it well, rinse it thoroughly, and allow it to completely air-dry. The potato should be fully mature and not in the green or early stages of development. Neither must it have begun to sprout or ever been frozen. It should also be free from toxic pesticides, weed killers, and other harmful chemicals.

For this particular poultice, the Cayce readings are fairly specific: *scrape*—do not peel—the skin of an *old* (not new) Irish potato with a kitchen knife or a fine-shredding grater. A small amount of the pulp can also be grated, making enough moisture to hold the mixture together. Separate into two piles, about one tablespoon each, and place each pile in a glass or china cup. Eyes should be free of makeup; contact lenses, if you are wearing them, should be removed.

Place the potato scrapings over closed eyes, making sure that the eye socket is filled with the moist, mushy material. Fasten it in place with gauze or a bandage, lean back in a reclining chair or lie down on a bed, and leave on from as little as ten minutes to as long as overnight. If

leaving it on overnight, a narrow band of cloth can be tied behind the
head. One reading advised applying the poultice *between* the gauze layers (2638-1).

After removing the poultice, the eye is bathed with a mild antiseptic,
such as a boric acid solution or a weakened Glyco–Thymoline application (one part Glyco to two parts distilled water). Use cotton balls (two
in small paper cups) to administer the cleanser. Cleaning the eyes after
a potato poultice avoids a localized infection and prevents reabsorption
of the toxins which have created the original condition and have been
drawn out by applying the poultice. It is critical, therefore, to wash the
eyes thoroughly after the potato poultice is removed. If the area feels
somewhat sticky from the antiseptic solution, use a wet washcloth or
dampened cotton balls to further bathe the eyes and clear up the stickiness.

DIRECTIONS FROM THE READINGS

For a forty–nine–year–old male suffering from retinitis pigmentosa
(reading given on December 22, 1930):

> . . . use those properties of the scraped Irish potato as an ointment over
> the eye itself. Be sure that the eye is closed, and use sufficient to fill
> the socket or indentation of eye itself, with a bandage put over same
> for the evening; or it may be taken off early in the morning. Following
> the removal of same, be sure that there is a cleansing of the eyes with
> a weakened solution as an antiseptic eyewash, see?   2-20

For a female adult (no age given), who according to eye specialists
had tuberculosis of the eyes (reading given on September 12, 1933):

> When there is any irritation of the lids and the eye itself, we would also
> use a poultice over the cavity of the eye made from scraped Irish po-
> tato; not new potatoes, however, neither those that have sprouted.
> Scrape them and use sufficient to fill the cavity of the eye, see? This
> would be applied at night and bound so that it would not cause trouble
> to the body. Of mornings, or if irritation arises later in the evening

(but should remain on all night when possible), cleanse the eye socket
and cavity with an antiseptic solution. This will tend to make for an
easing of the disturbed forces.   360-3

[She had trouble sleeping and would get up three or four times
throughout the night. Edgar Cayce in a letter suggested that she use the
potato poultice in the afternoons or evenings since it was too difficult
for her to leave it on overnight.]

For a forty–one–year–old male suffering from cataracts, which could
have resulted from an injury to the left eye (reading given on December
15, 1941):

> ... we would apply a scraped Irish potato poultice over the eyes; that is,
> scrape an *old* Irish potato (not new potato) and apply between gauze.
> Let this remain on the eye for at least thirty to forty minutes. Then
> bathe off the eyes (when this is removed) with a weak eye lotion, such
> as will remove some of the inflammation that is drawn by the potato.
> 2638-1

TESTIMONIALS/RESULTS

A report from Miss [4012] (February 15, 1950):

> "I used grated old Irish potatoes over my eyes several times daily and
> at night—it kept the condition {*conjunctivitis*} cleared up enough that
> I could continue work all summer. I have since taken allergy tests which
> showed up positive and am now taking injections. However, the pota-
> toes gave me the only relief in five years, but couldn't clear up the
> allergy—I hope the injections are the answer. I can understand how
> potatoes could permanently clear up some forms of conjunctivitis—
> but since my particular kind was an allergy, it had to be removed. But I
> thank God for the potatoes until I found the cause." 1963-1, Report #8

A report from Mrs. S.W. McComb (January 22, 1950):

"I have used the Irish potato poultice for my eyes with most pleasing results as it gave me the only relief from conjunctivitis I had. Before this I had the best of medical care with no relief. The condition of my eyes was most extreme and no permanent relief from treatments. With the Irish potato poultice I was much improved in three weeks. I kept the poultice on my eyes practically all night . . . About twice a year I use the potato poultice as a precaution. My eyes are now much better in every way."   1963-1, Report #7

A report from Mrs. Ruth Berkshire (September 23, 1960):

"When I was a little girl I picked up a beautiful case of what was later diagnosed as pink-eye. We lived twenty miles from town and doctor (a two-day round trip by horse and buggy) in a remote and rugged area of California. Morning after morning it was becoming more difficult for me to get my eyes 'unglued.' The day that I couldn't get them open and the grownups had to take over with a combination of worry, patience, washcloths, and warm water, some other adult was there and she (or he) suggested grinding up quite a few raw potatoes for a poultice to be tied over my eyes when I went to bed.

"I can well remember waking up still wearing my cold and clammy poultice and being able to open my eyes when it was removed and at how *good* my eyes felt. But I can't remember whether Mother repeated the treatment once more or not, but I do know that the potato poultice cleared up the infection practically overnight."   243-11, Report #4

A report from Bette Nelson, RN (November 19, 1973):

" . . . My mother, who was half Irish, raised five children on a farm and used no other treatment for anything except Irish potato poultices. We were never sick, and I never met a doctor till I was nineteen years old.

"Last year my friend's newborn baby contacted staph in the nursery, along with several others. I kiddingly told her to use the potato poultice. It cleared it up in three days. The infection was a severe one and not responding to any other medicine . . . "   5301-1, Report #6

ADDITIONAL INFORMATION

An ancient remedy, potatoes have been used in folk medicine in almost every country where they are grown, being applied to various parts of the body as needed. More than one hundred varieties of potatoes exist and, along with rice and wheat, the potato is one of the most important staple crops worldwide.

According to the U.S. Department of Agriculture, the potato is a near perfect food, supplying—when consumed with whole milk—almost all the food elements necessary for maintaining health in the human body. It is 99.9 percent fat free and is used as a dietary staple in over 130 countries.

The "birth" of the Irish white potato occurred about 4,500 years ago in the Andean Mountains of Peru and Bolivia, where it formed the basis of the Inca diet. Later, Spanish conquistadors arriving in Peru in the sixteenth century encountered this treasure, took them home, and from there potatoes spread throughout the world.

OTHER USES FOR THE POTATO

According to the Cayce readings, the skin—not the pulp—is the most nutritious and useful part of the potato. In addition to the scrapings used over the eyes, potato peelings were cooked in Patapar paper and the resulting juices were consumed like a soup as a dietary supplement. One twenty-five-year-old man was told that the peelings " . . . are strengthening, carrying those influences and forces that are active with the glands of the system . . . " (820-2)

Eating the peelings was also recommended to bring luster and restore color to the hair, to keep hair from graying, and to prevent hair from falling out. One thirty-three-year-old man asked about improving the growth of hair on his head. He was advised to eat not only potato skins, but also apple and apricot skins—cooked, not raw. " . . . these supply elements for the activity with the thyroids, that produce for the body the activities of the hair, the nails, and those portions of the system . . . " (826-1)

Lest we become too concerned about improving the quantity or quality of our head of hair, one reading also stated: "Don't worry about your hair. Worry about what you do with your mind and body. Let the hair, by the very activities, take care of itself. Those who do such, and worry about such, don't amount to much." (5190-1) Another individual was told: " . . . Brains and hair don't grow very well together at times anyway." (2301-5)

Potatoes, then, can be a beneficial addition to anyone's medicinal or dietary regimen.

Radio-Active Appliance

The name itself may deter some from using this remedy: "radio-active," yet that is how this appliance was named and described in the readings. Also called the Dry Cell, this device has no connection whatsoever with radioactivity, which became a household word after the 1945 destruction in Japan from the early atomic bombs. Possibly the appliance is comparable to a radio wave because of a vibrational current between it and the user. The Edgar Cayce Foundation suggested the name Impedance Device. Today it is known as Radiac® and is sold through A.R.E.'s official worldwide supplier.

A four-sided figure shaped slightly like a pyramid, this device is mentioned in over eight hundred Cayce documents. The six-inch-high dark-blue container with a red strip near its top holds carbon steel plates separated by glass panes and surrounded by blocks of carbon and coarsely ground charcoal. An instructional booklet for its care, use, and storage is included with each purchase. The appliance can be used as is (plain) or with a solution jar attached.

According to the readings, the Radiac® effects a change in the body's electrical energy by utilizing the body's own current. It looks like a battery but contains no electrical energy of its own. It does emit a subtle force often detected by sensitive individuals. The two terminals on the top of the appliance are each connected by a wire to an electrode or disc that is attached to the body. "Its design," according to Harvey Grady's article "A Gift on the Doorstep" (*Venture Inward*, May/June 1989, pp. 12-15), "creates a capacitor which theoretically modulates the current flowing from one part of the body to another." This equalizing effect is mentioned in several readings. Though the appliance was noted as good for everyone, certain specific instructions may need to be followed to obtain results. It is highly recommended that one read about the device (*see*, for example, the Circulating File on "Appliances: Radio-Active") before applying it. The device is used most often as a preventive rather than as a curative measure.

INDICATIONS

Alcoholism, anemia, appendicitis, arthritis, catarrh, cerebral palsy, circulatory incoordination, cold feet, colds, congestion, deafness, debilitation, digestive problems, enlarged joints or any protuberance, epilepsy, frequent and painful urination, goiter, hypertension, insomnia, intestinal disturbances, leukemia, menopause, menstrual cramps, menstrual irregularity, nausea, nervous tension and incoordination, neurasthenia, neuritis, obesity, poor memory, prenatal or reproductive conditions, rheumatism, senility, spinal subluxations, stress, torticollis, vaginitis, vision problems

CONTRAINDICATIONS

Maintain a positive mental attitude when using the device; do not use if in a negative mental or emotional state; since the device takes on the body's own energy and vibrations, no one else should use your appliance; do not use on the same day that you are taking sedatives or any kind of alcoholic beverage; do not use during the menstrual period; do not store the appliance in the refrigerator or on or near metal objects; do not use with other Cayce-related electrical appliances (such as the Violet Ray or the Wet Cell)

MATERIALS NEEDED
Radiac® device
Two small discs with loop straps and hooks (one positive red wire and one negative black wire)
Emery cloth sanding paper
Protector cap for the device
[The previous items are included in a Starter Kit.]
Large, deep plastic, glass, or ceramic bowl (nonmetal)—to fill with ice and set device in
Jumper wire
Solution jar with storage cap
Element wire assembly
Brush with handle
Extra-wide hook and loop belt
[The last five items are needed if you are using one solution; they are included and can be purchased in a Solution Jar Starter Set (which also comes with two discs and one negative and one positive wire).]
Solution—if using with the device (includes gold chloride, gold sodium, camphor, iodine, silver nitrate, or tincture of iron)

FREQUENCY OF APPLICATION
Daily; once or twice a day; may be done in cycles: example, 4-day sequence (see *Directions*)—may leave off 4 days to 1 week, then repeat 4-day sequence; once, 3, or 4 times each week; once a month; 30 days, rest 10 days, resume for 30 days; 3 weeks, rest 1 week, repeat for 3 weeks

LENGTH OF TIME OF APPLICATION
In the beginning about 10 minutes, gradually increasing each time up to 30 minutes (by the third or fourth time); 20 minutes in the beginning, gradually increasing by 5 minutes each day of treatment; in the beginning 30 minutes each day (may be increased to 60 minutes after 15 to 18 days); 30 minutes to 1 hour; 4 hours in each 24 hours (for 10 to 12 days), then reduce to 1 or 2 hours each evening

LOCATION OF APPLICATION

Plain—pulse points on wrists and ankles (rotated with each treatment)

With solution—various points: umbilicus and lacteal duct area, extremities, along spine (follow individual readings specific to your health concern)

WHEN TO USE THE RADIO-ACTIVE APPLIANCE

When feeling overanxious, overtired, mentally or physically taxed, distressed, in pain, needing relaxation or rest, just before retiring (bedtime)

EXPECTED EFFECTS/PURPOSES

Improves and equalizes circulation

Normalizes the functioning of the nervous system

Aids in relaxing the body and reducing stress

Helps with memory and meditation

Balances the vibratory rate in the extremities

Normalizes blood pressure, heart rate, and kidney functions

Stimulates the body and mind to better organize and integrate their functioning

Improves peripheral blood circulation

Attunes the vibrations of the body to an optimal state

Reduces blood impurities

Helps create a better metabolism

DIRECTIONS

Until one gets used to the procedure, it may seem daunting to hook up the Radio-Active Appliance with its discs, wires, and loop straps. But within a short time the task should become "second nature."

The appliance is placed in the sun for about an hour between uses (cloudy days are OK) in order to maintain the individual's own vibrations that build up within it over time. It may be placed on a windowsill next to nonmetallic window frames. Twenty minutes before you hook up to it, put the device into a plastic, glass, or ceramic (nonmetal) container (about a gallon-size) and fill the basin with ice up to the red strip, one-and-a-half inches from the top of the appliance, then add water to the same level. The ice and cold water help to "electronize" the device. While it's resting in this tub, clean the surfaces of the electrode discs by polishing them with a cloth, and then sand them lightly with emery paper. This removes the film buildup from the body's vibrations and prevents short-circuiting.

After twenty minutes with the device remaining in the ice water, connect first the red (positive) wire to the red jack on the appliance. Next, connect the black (negative) wire to the black jack, making sure that the discs do not touch each other. Lie down nearby and attach the red disc to your body, next, the black disc. (Notice that in connecting the wires to the jack and placing the discs on the body, you always start with the positive one.)

These electrodes are placed directly on the skin, attached with Velcro to maintain a firm contact but without inhibiting circulation. With each application they are rotated sequentially over the pulse points on the ankle (inner, big toe side) and wrist (thumb side of hand). Here are the recommended attachment positions of the discs for a four-day sequence (as noted earlier, "red" and "black" refer to the colors of the wires: red=positive, black=negative):

Day 1	right wrist (red)	left ankle (black)
Day 2	left wrist (red)	right ankle (black)
Day 3	left ankle (red)	right wrist (black)
Day 4	right ankle (red)	left wrist (black)

Notice the placement on opposite sides of the body. The (positive) red disc is always attached first. When removing the wires after use, *reverse the order.*

If you skip a day or two, make note of the position last used so that when you resume you will continue with the next position in the sequence. Though it takes four days to finish a cycle, it is recommended that the cycle be completed if you happen to miss a treatment. Even if you use the device twice in one day, you would still move the discs to the next position. In case you hook up the wires incorrectly or touch the discs together, just skip that treatment period, put the device in the sun, and continue the sequence later.

In using a solution jar, the placement is slightly different, and it's best to follow a specific reading related to your health condition for determining the positions of the discs.

The length of time for the application is about thirty minutes, at least in the beginning. While connected to the device, maintain a relaxed, meditative state—pray or listen to soothing, inspirational music. At the end of the time period, when disconnecting, reverse the order, removing first the black (negative) attachment from your body, then the red (positive) one. Next, remove the black wire from the appliance, followed by the red wire. Take the device out of the ice tub.

It is important to rest and relax for about thirty minutes after use, avoiding any excessive physical or mental activity, in order to allow the good results to continue. Keeping the black and red wires separated, clean and polish the discs as before and store them separately. The device, which has been removed from the ice container, may be placed in the sun for about an hour and then stored away from any metal objects. The solution jar, if used, is taken care of at this time. (The discs are cleaned and polished, as well as the loop that dips down into the solution jar.)

After completing the four-day sequence, you may stop using the device for four days to a week, and then resume the cycle again; or follow the directions as given in the specific reading you have chosen. More information is available in the booklet accompanying the kit.

DIRECTIONS FROM THE READINGS

For a thirty-three-year-old man with insomnia, catarrh, and circulatory incoordination (reading given on February 12, 1935):

> . . . each day for a period of a month at a time—thirty day periods and a rest period of ten days, then another thirty day period and then leaving it off for ten days, then another thirty day period—we would use those vibrations from the Radio-Active Appliance, to the opposite poles of the body, or extremities, each time it is applied. To the left wrist and right ankle, to the right wrist and the left ankle. This we would take preferably as the body rests just before retiring; and we will have little

or no disturbance with those tendencies for insomnia or for the keep-
ing awake.   826-1

A female (no age given) was suffering from poor circulation, headaches, and a tendency toward diabetes (reading given on October 16,
1935):

> . . . we would stimulate the normal circulatory force by the use of the
> Radio-Active Appliance. This will balance the circulatory forces in the
> nerve energies and blood supply, that will make for the soothing, as it
> were, of the whole of the nerve force; tending to make the rest more
> helpful.
> This we would take *each* day for thirty minutes to an hour, for three
> weeks. Then rest from same a week, and then take again. And then
> *whenever* there are the periods of overtiredness, overanxiety, the de-
> sire on the part of the body to make for real rest, use same—the Appli-
> ance.
> We would make the attachments alternately to the right wrist and
> left ankle, left wrist and right ankle—each time that it may be used,
> when using in periods; or rotary use . . .
> (Q) Any other suggestions for this body at this time?
> (A) With the use of the Radio-Active Appliance, if these are used as
> periods of concentration and meditation and prayer, the body will find
> that the experiences will bring a very helpful influence into the mental
> and spiritual life of the body.
> Be consistent, persistent with these things suggested.
> . . . Three weeks of the Radio-Active Appliance to begin with. And
> each week have the massage and rubs following the sweats. The sweats
> should be rather the cabinet sweats, and not too hot for the body but
> sufficient to cause the activity of the superficial circulation to form a
> portion of the eliminating forces.
> And these will make for bettered conditions for this body, [1022].
>   1022-1

For a twenty–two–year–old woman who was struggling with obesity (reading given on May 18, 1931):

> . . . While there is the tendency for the body to immediately take on
> weight when the diet is neglected, or too much sugars or too much
> starches are added to the system, we will find that were the vibrations
> added in the proper ratio or manner from the Radio-active Appliance
> (the plain), the assimilated forces will be better distributed in the sys-
> tem and the *vibrations* as are set up will be nearer *equalized,* and that
> conditions will then *continue* to be in a nearer *normal* way and man-
> ner; for *these* vibrations *now,* with the changes as have come about in
> system, will act with the *glands* of the system that tend to make for too
> much of the avoirdupois of body . . .
>
> With the application of the Radio-Active Appliance, these we would
> alternate from the opposite sides—rather than being opposite. When
> attached to the right wrist, attach to the right ankle. When attached to
> the left wrist, attach to the left ankle. See? . . .
>
> (Q) How often and how long at a period should the Radio-Active Appli-
> ance be used?
>
> (A) At least thirty minutes each day. This may be increased to sixty
> minutes when this has been taken for fifteen to eighteen days
>
> 2096-2

TESTIMONIALS/RESULTS

Two longtime Study Group members, Brent and Barbara Parisen, who
attended a Search for God group in Eastlake, Ohio, where they were
married, wrote about "Our Experiences with the Radio-Active Appliance" in *The A.R.E. Journal* (March 1978). Brent has a BS in electrical engi-
neering from the University of Michigan, and Barbara received her BA
in English from Cleveland State University. After describing the workings of the device, they note its physical and spiritual benefits:

> "With the very first application came immediate relaxation. We just
> wanted to curl up and go to sleep! . . . In fact, when we do sleep with the
> appliance attached, we sleep deeper and wake up fully rested and rar-
> ing to go!   (p. 67)

" . . . we feel more 'put together' inside—more 'in order.' There is a
wonderful sense of well-being, a deep, internal peace . . .   (p. 68)
"The appliance has improved our circulation. I especially have been
made aware of this, for there is more color in my face and I no longer
suffer with cold hands and feet . . .   (p. 68)

"Brent believes the machine has helped to correct his metabolism . . .
he has lost 17 pounds from his 5'11" frame without dieting and has
remained at the reduced weight of 158 pounds for the past six months.
                                                                (p. 68)

" . . . we have found since using it that our memories have improved.
We remember things at the most appropriate times; we don't have to
hunt mentally for the right words with which to express ourselves during conversations; we retain more of what we read; and we remember
our dreams more often and in greater detail.   (p. 68)

"Our dreams have become more lucid—often we know what the dream
means while dreaming it or immediately upon awakening.   (p. 68)

" . . . The balance brought about by the radio-active appliance seems to
have created a greater determination within us both to learn, to grow,
to overcome. We are possessed with a tremendous drive to work, to do
the things we must do, to do what He would have us do . . . This is
without doubt the greatest blessing brought to us through the use of
the radio-active appliance . . . "   (p. 69)

ADDITIONAL INFORMATION

Repeatedly recommended as "good for everybody," the Radio–Active
Appliance is unfortunately used by a relatively limited number of individuals. Just how it works still remains puzzling even though theories
related to subtle energies are presented.

Statements from the readings describe the workings of the appliance
as a *generative* magnet" (1800–28), which " . . . takes energies in portions
of the body, builds up and discharges body electrical energies that re-

vivify portions of the body where there is a lack of energies stored." (3105-1) The vibrations of the appliance " . . . are the lowest form of electrical forces that move as energies from the etheronic forces—or of the lowest form of static, or the electrical creative forces . . . " (681-2) Elsewhere the readings state: " . . . the lowest form of electrical vibration is the basis of life . . . " (444-2)

As mentioned earlier, anyone can benefit from its use, " . . . for the system would be improved in every condition that relates to the body being kept in attunement . . . " (1800-5) The Radiac® is said to equalize the body system's vibratory forces, producing rest and relieving nervousness, even though nothing may be felt while one is using it. The changes may come about gradually, making the body more physically and mentally fit " . . . to be of a greater service, to find more and greater opportunities for the expression of that gained . . . " (531-6)

How long will this "battery" last? Evidently it has a long life:

> The Active battery, when in *accord*—that is, all of the connections made properly, or kept so—is the life of the use of same; there's no ending. Is there an *ending* in life? an ending in vibration? It is *vibration* that is created.
>
> 5510-2

If your body is actually building the charge that will be disseminated by the appliance throughout your body, it would be important to be mindful of what you are creating. For this reason also, you should be the sole user of your device.

It is not to be used on the same day you are taking sedatives or alcoholic beverages. It is not to be stored in the refrigerator or on or near metal. Other cautions worth noting are:

> . . . This is beneficial to *anyone, properly* used! It is harmful, improperly used.
>
> You can't use the Radio-Active Appliance and be a good "cusser" or "swearer"—neither can you use it and be a good hater. For it will work as a boomerang to the whole of the nervous system if used in conjunction with such an attitude . . .
>
> 1844-2

Those building the appliance are also advised to observe the same caution, not constructing the device while they are angry, emotionally distressed, or upset. (See also *Contraindications*.)

For some physical conditions, a solution jar containing the medication is utilized as an additional attachment to the body. This jar provides a unique application of medication since its vibrations, rather than the compound itself, are introduced into the body. The readings suggest that the vibration from the solution stimulates the body, reminding it what it needs and enticing the body to produce it. For example, someone with anemia needs more iron in the blood, so it is possible that " . . . the addition of iron . . . adds, through this electronic atomic force, that same action in that portion of the system that creates that reaction . . . " (1800–15)

Solutions available on the market today include gold chloride, gold sodium, camphor, iodine, silver nitrate, and tincture of iron. Refer to the individual readings that deal with your particular health issue and follow the recommendations mentioned as to the type of solution, placement of the discs, and length of time of application.

Some comments from the readings on several of the solutions are included here as additional items of interest:

> (Q) . . . would the application of this {*tincture of iron*} cure anemia?
> (A) Cure anemia, even in a virulent or exaggerated state. This would of necessity be rather the preventive than curative forces, though with the application of this we gradually build that condition in the system to overcome, or add iron to the system, see?
> (Q) Would tincture of iodine cure goitre?
> (A) Tincture of iodine cures and prevents goitre. This, as we find, would reduce any condition that affects the ductless glands. Would also prove preventives, in cases first beginning, of appendicitis, or of any condition relating to either thyroid or the appendix.
> (Q) What would spirits of camphor, silver nitrate and gold chloride, each, cure?
> (A) Silver nitrate is a nerve stimulant, see? Any condition pertaining to the nerve system. Chloride of Gold . . . any condition wherein there

is any form of the condition bordering on rheumatics, or of the necessity of rejuvenating any organ of the system showing the delinquency
in action, see? Nitrate as is added through the silver solution to central portions (which may be alternated with gold and silver) for those
of a neurotic condition, even unto neuritis, or any form of condition
pertaining to enlarged joints, muscles, tissue, any protuberance as
comes to portions of body, see?

(Q) What would the spirits of camphor cure?

(A) Nausea and summer complaints. Any intestinal disturbance.

(Q) Would the system absorb the tincture of iron, or merely the vibration as given off by the tincture of iron?

(A) The vibration as given off, which creates that same vibration, giving the action with the elements in the system that create iron, those
properties or those actions of same in system . . . it would be beneficial
to all human force of life . . .   1800-6

One final note regards the reaction that some individuals may occasionally experience when using the appliance, especially in the beginning. The readings mention nausea, irritations, or worry—sometimes
due to the combining of the vibrations of metals in the system. These
reactions are often necessary for cleansing and balance and usually dissipate after only a few uses of the appliance.

Red Wine with Black Bread

If you ever need a "picker–upper" to get you through the afternoon doldrums, you may want to try a suggestion found in nearly eighty Cayce readings: a mid–afternoon separate meal consisting of a little red wine accompanied by black or brown bread.

As with many other dietary items in the readings, this combination of red wine with bread has a medicinal effect on the body. It is to be eaten *as a meal* with no other food—no cake, pastries, or sweets—just the wine and bread alone.

INDICATIONS

General debilitation, incoordination between assimilation and elimination, low immune system, poor appetite, toxemia, weakness, when needing a stimulant

CONTRAINDICATIONS

Use caution and moderation in relation to alcoholic beverages; the readings warn consistently against excessive amounts of drinks or foods that produce fermentation

MATERIALS NEEDED

Red wine, light wine, sherry, port, or "communion wine" (325-60); " . . . taken . . . as food, *not* as drink." (849-19); not white or sour wine (vinegar) or wine that is too sweet

Black or brown bread (pumpernickel, sour or heavy bread, rye, whole wheat—sometimes toasted or as wafers—or Ry-Krisp)—small slice

FREQUENCY OF APPLICATION

Daily, once a day, 2 or 3 times a week

DOSAGE

Small glass of red wine, sipped slowly; 1 or 2 ounces; ½ jigger or 1 jigger (1 jigger equals about 1½ fluid ounces) up to 2½ ounces; half a wine glass; full small wine glass

WHEN TO TAKE THE WINE AND BREAD

Mid-afternoon; around 2, 3, 4, or 5 o'clock in the afternoon; between noon and evening meals; " . . . about thirty minutes to an hour or so before the evening meal . . . " (1898-1); "cocktail time" (578-5, 849-13); late afternoon; evenings; " . . . when first returning from activity . . . " (357-12); soon after or with beef juice; " . . . three or four days after the cleansing of the system . . . " (1898-1)

LENGTH OF TIME OF APPLICATION

Take regularly; take for 10 days, off a few days, then resume

EXPECTED EFFECTS/PURPOSES

Has a stimulating reaction on the digestive system
Is " . . . laxative in its *reaction* . . . " (1192-6)
Tones the digestive forces
Assists the assimilation of food
Is blood- and body-building
Builds resistance in the glandular system
Absorbs poisons from the system
Has a strengthening effect on the body

DIRECTIONS

Around two to five o'clock in the afternoon, thirty minutes to an hour before the evening meal, sit down and relax for a small "meal" of red wine and black (or brown) bread. The wine may be a full, small wine glass, one-half of a glass, or one to two-and-a-half ounces in amount. Sip it slowly, without gulping it; and take it as a food and not as a drink, the readings say.

The bread accompanying the wine—either black or brown, whole wheat wafers or Ry-Krisp—is a small slice and may even be dunked into the wine, if you prefer. This is a meal—not a snack—to be eaten slowly and sipped unhurriedly. No other food items are to be taken with this combination—no pastries, sweets, cakes, and the like—simply the bread and wine.

DIRECTIONS FROM THE READINGS

For a thirty-six-year-old woman suffering from stomach lacerations, poor eliminations, and indigestion (reading given on August 12, 1937):

> No strong drinks or any food that makes for a quantity of alcohol in its activity in the system; that is, no cocktails, no beer. Wine may be taken *as* a food, not as a drink. Red Wine in the late afternoon is very well, not more than an ounce and a half to two ounces; preferably with black or brown bread.   1422-1

A forty-three-year-old man had a nervous stomach and incoordination between his assimilations and eliminations (reading given on May 28, 1939):

> Of late afternoons when first returning home, we find that red wine as a food—not as a drink—would be very strengthening, and well for the body. This would be taken only with black or brown bread; about two ounces each afternoon—about thirty minutes to an hour or so before the evening meal—would be materially aiding to the body. This should not be begun, though, until three or four days after the cleansing of the system is accomplished.   1898-1

A forty–nine–year–old male with anemia and general debilitation as well as assimilation and elimination incoordination (reading given on November 8, 1939):

> As we find, in bringing about those things that may help or aid in bringing better conditions for this body, it will take *persistence* and patience, *and* the correct diet; though this may at times appear to be rather severe upon the body, and the refraining from any of alcoholic drinks of any nature—save at times, in the late afternoon (three or four or five o'clock), the red wine may be taken if it is taken as a food; that is, as sort of a booster in the late afternoon, with only about an ounce and a half to two ounces taken with *only* a small slice of brown or pumpernickel bread with same.   2039-1

TESTIMONIALS/RESULTS

Mrs. [954], thirty–eight years old, wrote a letter to Cayce on March 21, 1936, remarking on suggestions and phrases from her reading. Here is an account of her comments and Cayce's subsequent reply:

> " . . . how is Mr. Hearst {*William Randolph Hearst (1863-1951), US editor and publisher*} going to feel when he sees us reeling in to knock off a bit of copy having had our glass of red wine in the middle of the business day? It is our opinion that Mr. Hearst is going to say . . . 'If you can't keep sober on the job, [954] . . . ' And we leave the rest to your morbid imagination . . . "   954-2, Report #2

Cayce responded three days later:

> " . . . As for the red wine, maybe you'll have to defer that until *after* office hours—just so it is an hour or hour and a half before dinner. You'll just have to wait a bit later to eat your dinner . . . "
>
>   954-2, Report #3

On March 27, 1950, Mrs. [264] replied to a questionnaire regarding her readings from Cayce:

"Have taken 1 to 2 ounces of red wine with whole wheat wafers, or 1 slice of whole wheat bread, to build red cells. This was taken about 4 p.m. (Virginia Dare Red Wine—Garrett's) Blood count proved this to have been beneficial.

"The above taken for a few weeks brought about an improvement in blood count, as well as in my digestion! . . . "   264-32, Report #6

Mrs. [5211] wrote a report on May 15, 1940, about her treatments, mentioning her use of the wine and bread combination:

" . . . I assume whole wheat bread can be substituted for the black bread suggested with the red wine. Black bread not available. I have mostly avoided bread altogether, even whole wheat. But recently, have started taking an ounce of Port wine and a thin slice of whole wheat bread toasted daily. Perhaps it will aid in energy pick up. Am using this between meals, assuming it should not be taken with other foods."

5211-1, Report #17

ADDITIONAL INFORMATION

What effect does this combination of wine and bread have on one's body? Several readings mention its stimulating reaction, especially on the digestive system, as well as its strengthening effect. One reading notes that copper, iron, and silicon are the " . . . blood–building properties that come from such a combination—especially at this hour {mid-afternoon} . . . " (1014-1) Another reading states that " . . . the absorption of {red wine} by the nature of the bread indicated {black or brown}, and sipped, makes for an absorbing of poisons from the system rather than creating those conditions that produce fermentation, see? . . . " (1044-1)

One woman was told that taken in the late afternoon red wine with black bread was "much more preferable" than coffee or tea, plus " . . . it doesn't put on weight, it doesn't make for souring in the stomach . . . " (1073-1) (See also *Expected Effects/Purposes*.)

When asked about taking intoxicating drinks, Cayce told one person: "*Wine* is good for all, if taken alone or with black or brown bread . . . not too much—and just once a day. Red wine only." (462-6)

What did Cayce mean by red wine? A forty–eight–year–old man received this answer:

> Means *red* wine! Not white wine, not sour wine; not that that is too
> sweet but any of those that are in the nature of adding to the body the
> effect of grape sugar.
>
> There is a variation, to be sure, in the character of sugars and the
> necessary forces and influences of that carried on in the system in
> producing assimilation.
>
> Foods must ferment, naturally, from acid, the action of acid and
> alkalin{*e*}. These passing into the duodenum {*first section of the small
> intestine*}, especially, become then certain characters of sugars; as pro-
> duced by the activity of the pancreas juices upon the effect of juices
> from the liver and the spleen, in digestive forces.
>
> Then the addition of Red wine, which is carrying more of a tartaric
> effect upon the active forces of the body, is correct; while those that
> are sour or that draw out from the system a reaction upon the
> hydrochlorics become detrimental.   437-7

[Tartaric acid is a clear, colorless, crystalline acid found in vegetable
tissues and fruit juices.]

The relationship of fermentation of foods to the acids in one's body
is explained in this way. While red wine was definitely to be consumed
for the afternoon "meal," other wines, such as " . . . the sauterne or the
light wines . . . should always be *with* meals, not separate." (1192–6) For at
least six individuals, no mention was made of including bread, only
that the wine was to be taken. Advice recommending this duo was
generally given in the context of dietary suggestions or the result of
questions about the advisability of taking intoxicating drinks or liquors.

Sand Pack

The sand pack is one remedy that would not qualify as a "home" remedy—unless you live near the beachfront! Yet those who enjoy sunbathing *on* the beach may also enjoy lying *in* the sand, a treatment referred to in the Cayce readings as a "sand pack."

Many people, after spending some time in Virginia Beach, VA, learn that the sand there is special. A twenty-four-year-old woman suffering from chronic ulcerative colitis was informed that " . . . The radiation from the gold and radium in the proportions that you find in Virginia Beach . . . is the better for the conditions of the body." (5237-1) Of course, it wasn't the type of gold to attract a "forty-niner's" gold rush as in California, but the sand was beneficial enough to entice participants to receive a proper sand pack when they visited Virginia Beach. Many A.R.E. conferees throughout the years have participated in this treatment as part of their overall conference experience.

Sand packs were mentioned in fifty-nine readings for thirty-seven individuals. Virginia Beach is not the only location for sand packs. Besides the Virginia coast, the west coast of Florida and, more specifically, the Clearwater and St. Petersburg, FL, areas are also good locations. Seabreeze Beach is noted, but its exact location is not given. One mention is made of each of the following: the east coast of Florida, the lower coasts of California, and the beaches of North Carolina. When asked if salt water was beneficial, Cayce answered that the "Sand that carried gold and radium and salt . . . " was the most beneficial. (3868-1)

INDICATIONS

Adhesions, anemia, arthritis, cerebral palsy, colitis, eczema, epilepsy, general debilitation, head noises, incoordination of nervous systems, lesions, lumbago, neurasthenia, neurosis, poor circulation, poor eliminations, retinitis, sluggish liver, spinal subluxations, toxemia, tuberculosis, tumors

CONTRAINDICATIONS

Use caution with heart or circulatory problems or high blood pressure (may be too hard on the heart or too stimulating); claustrophobia; do not use the ultraviolet light with sand packs (2-12)

MATERIALS NEEDED

Section of dry sand on beach
Swimsuit
Sand pails and shovels—to prepare area for lying down
Towel, umbrella, or porous hat—to provide shade and/or cover the face

FREQUENCY OF APPLICATION

Daily; every other day; daily for 1 week or 10 days; 3 to 5 days in a row; 1, 2, 3, or 4 times a week; for 4 or 5 days; frequency depends upon reaction of the body and the weather

LENGTH OF TIME OF APPLICATION

Five to 8 minutes; 10 to 15 to 20 to 30 minutes, then afterwards rest 15 to 20 minutes; 20 to 30 minutes; 30 to 60 minutes

LOCATION OF APPLICATION

Around knees, ankles, sciatic center, and ileum plexus; lower limbs (thighs, legs, feet); arms (upper, lower, hands); torso; leave uncovered the face—mouth and eyes

TIME OF DAY FOR SAND PACK

Never between 10:30 a.m. and 2:30 p.m.; appropriate times: 9 to 10 a.m. or 3 to 4 p.m.; early morning or late evening

EXPECTED EFFECTS/PURPOSES

Benefits the general nervous system

Helps body to absorb iodine

Builds up the blood and nerve systems

Clarifies and stimulates blood flow, especially in lungs and liver

Stimulates the capillary circulation

Produces a " . . . quickening, or pulsation through the superficial circulation . . . " (849-41)

DIRECTIONS

The Cayce readings are clear and specific in explaining the procedure for a sand pack. First, the sand that is to cover you must be dry and warm. Even if there has been a rainfall of short duration, the underlying sand where the body is to be partially buried may still be moist and cool and, therefore, not appropriate for use. One may have to wait several days, then, for the deeper layers of sand to dry out.

If the deeper sand is dry, take a dip in the ocean first, enveloping yourself entirely with sea water (this will help with iodine absorption). " . . . Dip under like you are being baptized properly!" (264-46) Then, immediately cover yourself or get someone to cover you with the dry, warm sand. Afterward, one person was told, " . . . {follow} same by a fresh bath and a spirited rubdown along the spine . . . ." (421-4) Another was told to rest " . . . for fifteen to twenty minutes, at *least, so that* the body has the *opportunity* to *respond to* those vibrations set up; for the pulsation is *equalized* by such applications . . . " (758-18) The sand pack treatment may also be concluded by a quick dip in the ocean.

Packers and recipients remain quiet and reverent throughout the treatment. Duties of the packers include preparing the area of the beach for the recipient: obtaining pails of extra sand from along the dunes, "... that which has not been trampled over too much ... " (849-37), and digging out the sand where the person would lie down. Level the sand in an east-west direction, making small sand pillows to support the back of the neck and under the knees. " ... at first {cover} only the lower limbs and the upper limbs, the arms and legs. Then gradually more and more cover the whole body, keeping the face in shadow or in the shade ... " (264-46) Covering the recipient with sand is to be done with an attitude of love and caring.

Excluding the face and head, the rest of the body should be in the sun as much as possible. Packers continue to monitor the person, removing any sand from an area that feels too heavy or uncomfortable and helping the person up when the session feels complete. Afterward, the person rinses off in the nearby ocean.

DIRECTIONS FROM THE READINGS

For a thirty-one-year-old man with arthritis (reading given on November 25, 1938):

> When there is the sand and sea bath, it is well that the body be covered with sand afterward—dry sand. Let the body be thoroughly wet in the sea water—this meaning with the bathing suit and the body thoroughly wet—and then immediately cover the body in *dry* sand, see? not wet. Cover the entire body except, of course, the head and face— which should be shaded from the sun, while the rest of the body should be in the sun as much as possible—that is, the mound of sand *over* the body should be in the sun, see? Do not let there be such a weight on the body as to cause a great deal of distress by the weight of the sand, but let the body remain covered in this manner for twenty to thirty minutes, if it can be fairly comfortable for that length of time without it being a dread or a burden ...   849-33

For a forty-four-year-old woman with uterine tumors (reading given on July 3, 1935):

... And now under these existent conditions where there may be the applications from the activity of the actinic rays {*the chemically active rays, such as violet and ultraviolet parts of the spectrum*} of the sun and sand, these should be very effective to making for the addition in the physical reactions for the eliminations of much of the disturbances ...

First wet the body in the salt water, you see. Then let the body be covered almost entirely with *dry* sand; not wet sand but *dry* sand. Gradually, though, should this be done; that is, at first it would be only the lower limbs and the upper limbs, the arms and legs. Then gradually more and more cover the whole body; keeping the face in shadow or in the shade so that the reactions are not disagreeable. The pulsation caused by such activities is what we need. And do not keep in this too long in the beginning. For five to eight minutes at first. After a few days or a week, then increase it to ten to fifteen to twenty minutes. These should be of very great assistance.   264-46

TESTIMONIALS/RESULTS

Only a few references to sand packs appear in the Reports section of the readings, largely mentioning the application was followed. Herbert Avrum Levine, who worked at the A.R.E. in Virginia Beach as a massage therapist, Tai Chi instructor, and security guard, also assisted individuals with their sand pack experiences, particularly during conferences. Nicknamed "the Sandman," he drew up instructions and guidelines in June of 1982, teaching others how to give and receive sand packs. He also observed the results of their treatments.

Anecdotally, a number of individuals reported being free of joint pain. One woman even had a cessation of Ménière's syndrome (a malfunction of the semicircular canal of the inner ear) following her sand pack experience. Another woman, a smoker, mentioned the dark gray discoloration of the sand covering her chest area. The darkened sand showed up as the sand pack was being removed and indicated to her the release of toxins from her lungs. Other individuals noted how relaxed and balanced they felt after their sand pack treatment.

ADDITIONAL INFORMATION

Following is an excerpt from a letter written by Edgar Cayce, dated August 2, 1934, to Mr. [2483], discussing the benefits and formation of the Virginia Beach sand. Mr. [2483], a fifty–six–year–old real estate broker in Brooklyn, NY, requested a physical reading for a woman friend with sciatica. Cayce continues his letter:

" . . . Regarding her condition, sciatica, I would like to say that quite a number of physicians have sent such patients to Virginia Beach—even from Johns Hopkins and Mayo's—for recuperation. The sands here contain a great deal of radium and gold, which properties are quite beneficial in such conditions. And people get much help from just taking the sand baths on the seashore, to say nothing of other curative measures that might be added from here. The seashore here is quite a bit different from anywhere else in this respect; not that we have a sick colony, but a great many people from all over the country do come here for their health as much as for a summer resort. In fact, as a matter of record you will find that before the War {*World War I*} the Germans had obtained a permit to build a hospital at Virginia Beach—and for this very reason, on account of the great amount of beneficial properties in the sands along the seashore here. So, there is a condition here that exists in very few places in the world. The streams in the oceans run away from the land. The Gulf Stream coming up from the Florida coast and the Arctic Stream coming down unite opposite the Chesapeake Bay and turn across the ocean. Deposits both from the north and south are among the sands on the seashore at Virginia Beach, and you don't find such a condition anywhere else. Therefore, I believe it would do Mrs. [. . .] good; also we might be able to help her through information that we might obtain. Although we have no hospital in operation here at the present time (it having been closed since the beginning of the Depression), we do have the cooperation of several physicians in Virginia Beach and quite a number in Norfolk; so that, should Mrs. [. . .] require any special attention from any of these we would be able to obtain it for her . . . "   2483-2, Report #2

Showers

While many of us take showers automatically on a regular basis for hygienic purposes, we probably don't often consider this part of our routine as having a healing, therapeutic value. It might even be surprising to learn that showers were recommended as part of a regimen of treatment in the Cayce readings, usually sandwiched between a bath (such as, an Epsom salts bath or a steam/fume bath) and a massage.

By definition, a shower is a type of bath in which one's body is sprayed with heavy or fine streams of water at differing pressures and temperatures. Generally the water originates from an apparatus with a perforated nozzle that helps control the amount and variety of the mist or spray. This fixture is often attached overhead or, for a different effect, may be installed around the sides of the shower stall. Mentioned more than one hundred times in the health readings, showers remain a notable part of one's healing regimen.

INDICATIONS
Depression, eye discoloration, fatigue, general debilitation, head-aches, hernia, hypertension, joint pain, melancholia, menstrual

cramps, nervous system incoordination, poor circulation (blood and lymph), rashes, stress, toxemia

CONTRAINDICATIONS
Undue sensitivity or allergy to cold; no cold showers close to menstrual periods—take them at other times (1306-1); those with severe diabetes, impaired peripheral circulation, or cardiac problems may want to avoid cold applications or seek the advice of a physician

MATERIALS NEEDED
Access to a shower facility—bath tub, shower stall, etc.

Ability to control and regulate water temperature and pressure with faucet or dials

Coarse towels—used to rub down the body afterward

FREQUENCY OF APPLICATION
Daily, occasionally, once or twice a week, every morning, mornings and evenings, weekly, 3 to 4 times each week, every 10 days, take a " . . . cold shower as soon as the body steps out of bed {mornings} . . . " (342-3), 2 or 3 times a month

TEMPERATURE OF APPLICATION
Begin with tepid water, adding cold water gradually; alternate hot and cold water

LENGTH OF TIME OF APPLICATION
Have 3 to 5 to 10 or 12 to 14 treatments; for 3 weeks, rest 1½ to 2 weeks, then repeat; weekly for 6 to 8 weeks; 10 to 12 weeks; once every 10 days for 2 to 4 periods

LOCATION OF APPLICATION
Along and on the spine, whole body

WHEN TO TAKE THE SHOWER
After exercise, recreation, or sunbathing; after a colonic, a salt rub, or

a sand pack; before or after a steam/fume cabinet bath; after using the Wet-Cell Appliance; close to one's menstrual period; after a few osteopathic adjustments; after completing Atomidine series; evening before a workout (470-36); before using the Violet Ray device; before a massage

EXPECTED EFFECTS/PURPOSES

Stimulates superficial circulation

Relaxes and invigorates the body

Aids in coordinating and setting up eliminations and in removing poisons

Helps severe menstrual cramping to cease

Removes " . . . the necessity of taking stimulants to increase the blood cell forces . . . " (480-8)

Creates a " . . . much better appetite or an appetizing effect for the whole activity of the body." (714-2)

Cleanses the body following a steam/fume bath

DIRECTIONS

No specific instructions for showers are given in the readings, only the general direction to start with a warm, tepid shower and end with a gradual cooling, to alternate hot and cold water temperature, or simply to take a cold or hot shower.

In the first instance begin with a temperature that seems comfortable to you—what you usually bathe in. Then slowly add cold water until you reach a tolerable cool temperature. Allow yourself to soak in the spray for a short length of time. If you are taking the shower on a daily or almost daily basis, lengthen the time period as well as change the degree of temperature to a gradually colder setting. You will be surprised how after a few days or weeks you can become acclimated to a fairly cool temperature, one that you had previously found to be difficult to handle.

When positioned under the cool shower, allow the spray of water to fall onto your spine, covering that area. Then turn the water off, get a bath towel, hold it lengthwise at each end, and rub your back briskly with a back-and-forth motion, as if you are trying to dry it off. One reading described this as a " . . . rub-off of the cold . . . " (877-13) Finally, dry off your whole body and prepare for your massage.

A variation on this procedure is offered by Dr. Harold Reilly in his book *The Edgar Cayce Handbook for Health Through Drugless Therapy.* Once the water in the shower is warm, turn away from the shower nozzle and let it flow over your lower back. Next, bend over and slowly back into the shower stream, allowing it to hit the rest of your back. Gradually increase the warm setting up to a tolerable level—for about three to five minutes. Then quickly turn on the cold, letting the water hit the warm areas of your body. Count to forty, slowly. Turn the water off, wrap up in a large towel or robe, and relax in bed for ten minutes. Then dry off slowly, dress, and continue with your day. This long, hot shower followed by a cool quick one is very stimulating to circulation. Metabolism is speeded up and your body actually becomes warm. Avoid going out into cold weather immediately afterward. If you must go out, follow the first procedure with the slow warm and slow cool shower. This way the heat will be conducted away from the body without the metabolism's being affected too drastically. Remember: slow and cool—concludes Dr. Reilly.

A few readings advise the individual to take merely a cold or a hot shower; in some readings, no temperature is specified. Several others suggest alternating hot and cold water, such as the following: " . . . When ready to retire, give first the shower of hot and cold water—one, then the other, several times, to get this shock that comes from such sudden changes to the exterior of the body . . . " (1842-2) Again no details are given as to the exact procedure; however, hydrotherapy texts usually suggest a slightly longer time under the hot shower and a briefer time under the cold water. One also begins with heat and ends with cold. (For more information *see* the section **Alternating Hot and Cold** in the chapter "Cold and Hot Packs.")

DIRECTIONS FROM THE READINGS

For an adult woman with hypertensive tendencies and toxemia (reading given on April 10, 1943):

Do have occasionally a hydrotherapy treatment. This should include a mild sweat and then a thorough rubdown. Following the sweat there should be a hot and then a cold shower, to stimulate the superficial circulation. This, properly given, will aid in preventing further disturbance in the heart area, and that tendency for the blood pressure to be disturbing.   573-7

For a twenty–nine–year–old woman with nervous system incoordination (reading given on January 16, 1937):

(Q) Is it well for me to take cold showers in the morning?
(A) Better if they are taken tepid and gradually turned to cold. But whenever there is taken a cold shower, there should be a very, very brisk rubdown with coarse towels afterwards, especially along the spine.   808-5

For a thirty–four–year–old male with acidity problems, hypertension, toxemia, and lesions (reading given on March 11, 1941):

After the third osteopathic treatment—then we would have a full hydrotherapy treatment. This would include first a good, hot shower; then a cabinet bath; then a colonic irrigation; and then a shower with hot and cold water, followed by a thorough massage—especially using Peanut Oil along the spine, all that the body will absorb. Then have the rubdown, of course, with alcohol.   2462-1

For a nine-year-old girl, whose mother asked for directions in guiding her since, according to a letter dated September 28, 1934, her "mind seems strong" but " . . . the muscles fail to coordinate with the mind as well as we think they should . . . " (714-1, Background #1), and who was also suffering from malnutrition (reading given on March 5, 1935):

There should be also of mornings the warm or tepid bath, with a cold shower afterward, and a brisk rubdown especially along the spine. This should be adhered to; for these sudden changes or these conditions will prevent a great deal of this tendency towards languidness, as well as creating much better appetite or an appetizing effect for the whole activity of the body.   714-2

TESTIMONIALS/RESULTS

A forty-eight-year-old woman with poor circulation and poor elimi-nations was present for her physical reading on August 5, 1938. Two months later she wrote to Edgar Cayce:

> " . . . about the hot and cold water which I get at {*Dr. Harold*} Reilly's. I am the strangest person in that for the last three years or so (since I began ailing) I have not been able to have a hot or warm bath. Always cold. After I had had the reading and it spoke of the hot and cold water I thought I would try first hot and then cold when I had my shower. Well, immediately I started to have the sniffles and from then on the cold developed which ended in grippe. After I was completely over the grippe, I told Mr. Reilly about it and he says they {*staff at the Reilly Health Institute*} would regulate it so that the hose that was supposed to be hot was turned down to lukewarm, and so that is the only way I can take it. Even so, I get the sniffles and feel quite stirred up after the treatment—it seems to start things going in the sinuses, etc. How-ever, I think it is doing its work of helping the circulation, so I will continue but will do exactly as the reading says, twice a month and not oftener . . . "   1468-5, Report #3

Mr. [3428], a forty-four-year-old highway engineer with epilepsy who worked for the N.Y. State Highway Department, wrote to Cayce on Janu-ary 6, 1944, three days after receiving his reading:

> " . . . you mention 'needle shower.' I know what a needle shower is— but few homes have one, and I wondered whether an ordinary shower bath would suffice—or whether I could use an ordinary bath spray in-stead—that is—a regular head of a shower, and spray the water upon my body from different angles, while I am taking my shower. I can ap-preciate what better effects might be obtained through the use of a

needle shower—that is—to invigorate or stimulate the nerves, etc . . . ."   3428-1, Report #1

(See *Additional Information.*)

Two days later he wrote a follow-up letter in which he summarized Cayce's recommended regimen: " . . . after the sweat, I take a shower to wash myself clean—then use the *cold* water for the needle shower. After all this—then the massage." (3428-1, Report #2) In his letter he requested more information, but there is no record of Cayce's response.

ADDITIONAL INFORMATION

The term *needle shower* has nearly fifty mentions in the readings. At times it was given as an alternate shower bath in that the person could take a hot and cold shower or a needle shower (sometimes called a needle spray). This type of shower was available on the market in the late 1880s. The bather is surrounded by pipes that are exposed and visible alongside the walls or floor. A series of holes or openings lets out the water spray so that when it is in use, one becomes showered with water from all angles.

In hydrotherapy the terms *hot* and *cold* relate to normal oral body temperature: 98.6°F (37°C) with some fluctuations above or below these figures. A water temperature range of 100° to 104°F (38° to 40°C) is considered hot; tepid water ranges from 80° to 92°F (27° to 33°C); cold is 55° to 70°F (13° to 21°C). Depending upon where you live and the season of the year you're in, water temperature from cold pipes may be as low as 50°F (10°C) or as high as 70°F (21°C). Differences in water temperature allow for the creation of different effects in one's body.

Heat is relaxing, tepid is very relaxing, and cold is stimulating and energizing. Because a hot shower can also be tiring or fatiguing, the usual suggestion is for it to be followed by a short cold shower, just as the readings recommend. Cold water constricts and contracts whatever it hits, so even several seconds up to a minute or two of a cold shower may be extremely stimulating.

Over one hundred years ago, Father Sebastian Kneipp (1821–1897) maintained that taking regular cold showers would have a "hardening" effect on a person, boosting the body's defense system and thus preventing infection. In 1990, the Hanover Medical School in Germany decided to "retest" his claim. The six-month trial involved fifty medical students. Twenty-five students followed the Kneipp method of taking an early morning shower with increasing coldness, until in approximately three weeks they were taking two-to-three-minute cold showers each day. The remaining twenty-five students took only warm early morning showers throughout the test period. (If the students taking cold showers developed a cold, they immediately discontinued the cold application for one week and then resumed.)

For the first three months there was very little difference between the two groups: the number of colds contracted, their intensity, and their duration were about the same. But in the last three months these changes were noted: the cold-shower students had half the number of colds compared to the warm-shower group; also, their colds lasted half as long and were far less acute. Father Kneipp, it seemed, was correct.

While studying for the seminary, Kneipp contracted tuberculosis. Reading a booklet on the water cure, he decided to try it out on himself. Despite the wintertime temperatures, he bathed two or three times a week for a few minutes in the nearby Danube River. The following year, his health improved, and he entered the seminary to follow his lifelong dream of becoming a priest. During his priesthood, Father Kneipp continued his water ministry, treating poor and rich alike. His popular book, *My Water-Cure*, was widely translated; and his system, which included some 120 different types of water application, is taught and applied throughout Europe today.

Accordingly, you may want to consider showering for its therapeutic value. If possible, take a steam/fume bath before the shower and have a massage afterward. You will note the invigorating effects offered by this beneficial trio.

Sitz Bath

The term *sitz bath* comes partially from the German *Sitzbad*, meaning literally "sitting bath," in which the person sits immersed in water up to the waist in a tub shaped like a chair or large sink. Alternately, it is a basin over which the client squats to expose the lower external area to the steam rising from the water. Taking a sitz bath may also denote soaking in one's own bathtub. Whether one is immersed in water or sitting over the water, both types are mentioned in ninety of Cayce's readings. According to the degree of temperature, sitz baths may be cold, prolonged cold, neutral, very hot, a revulsion sitz bath, or alternating hot and cold (see *Directions*). Cayce recommended hot, tepid, and alternating. Sometimes substances, such as Epsom salts, tincture of myrrh, pine oil, or aloe, were added to the water. (*See also* the chapter on "Myrrh.")

INDICATIONS

Arthritis; constipation; cystitis; dysmenorrhea; eliminations incoordination; fatigue; fistulas; flu; grating knee and hip bone; hemorrhoids (use salt water); itching on thighs, legs, and vulva; menopause; nephritis; pelvic disorders; poor circulation; pregnancy; prostatitis;

pruritus; sterility; stiffness in joints and extremities; toxemia; tuberculosis (bone); vaginal irritations; venereal disease

CONTRAINDICATIONS

Never take a cold sitz bath if you feel cold or chilled; warm up by exercising, placing your feet in a basin of warm water, lying under blankets in bed, or taking a hot sitz bath—wait until you feel warm enough to take a cold sitz bath; otherwise, refrain from taking it

MATERIALS NEEDED

Basin, large bowl, or tub—to sit in or to sit over

Blanket, sheet, or large towel—to place around the shoulders and cover the upper body

Towels—to place around the basin or tub

Bowl of cold water and two washcloths—for cold compresses to neck and forehead (in neutral or hot bath)

Epsom salts (if used)—1 tablespoon of salt per one gallon of water

FREQUENCY OF APPLICATION

Occasionally; every second or third day; once or twice a week; every other week; 2, 3, or 4 times each week for 3 to 4 weeks; once or twice a month

LENGTH OF TIME OF APPLICATION

Sit over steam 5 to 8 minutes or 20 to 30 minutes; alternating hot, then cold 10 to 15 minutes for each; sometimes combined with a foot bath; often followed by massage

LOCATION OF APPLICATION

Body sits in waist-deep water in tub; for basin of hot water, steam is allowed to rise and to cover lower pelvic area while client squats over basin

AMOUNT OF DOSAGE

Tub sitz bath—1 tablespoon of Epsom salts per 1 gallon water; 6 to 9 inches of water in bathtub

WHEN TO TAKE SITZ BATH

Evenings; at rest time; 2 to 5 days prior to menstruation (for 2 to 3 months), but not just before or after menstrual flow; prior to or after spinal adjustments

EXPECTED EFFECTS/PURPOSES

Relieves congestion in lower abdomen

Relaxes the lumbar (lower spine) area

Reduces swelling and irritation from hemorrhoids

Coordinates lymph circulation

Relieves itching on thighs, legs, and vulva

Produces " . . . an expression to the nerve or that received through the sensory nervous system." (3771–1)

Aids in disturbances in rectal area

Induces relaxation

Helps to balance the body system

Makes " . . . for greater improvement through the lower portions of the locomotions, and the locomotion activities." (633–10)

DIRECTIONS

According to directions requested as guidelines from Dr. Harold J. Reilly on September 20, 1934 (which Gladys Davis often enclosed with a copy of the person's reading), the sitz bath tub may be an ordinary washtub or a tub made of porcelain or metal. A foot basin may be placed outside or inside the tub, whichever position is more comfortable, so that the feet can also be immersed in hot water. The temperature of this foot bath, however, should be at least two or three degrees above that of the sitz bath. The one receiving the bath can wrap a large towel, blanket, or sheet around him– or herself, with a cold–water compress applied to the head. For protection from contact with the tub, various towels can be placed under one's knees or behind one's back. Following are listed the specific procedures (appended to reading 3104–1) as described by Dr. Reilly for each type of sitz bath:

COLD SITZ BATH

Temperature: 55°F (12.7°C) to 75°F (23.8°C). Foot bath: 105°F (40.5°C) to 110°F (43.3°C). Length of time: 1 to 8 minutes or 2 to 4 minutes. Rub the hips to promote a reaction, using friction mitts, if desired. Greatly stimulates pelvic circulation.

PROLONGED COLD SITZ BATH

Temperature: 70°F (21.1°C) to 85°F (29.4°C). Foot bath: 105°F (40.5°C) to 110°F (43.3°C). Length of time: 15 to 40 minutes. (May begin at higher temperature and gradually lower it.) Should not cause chill; if warmth is needed, apply a hot-water bottle to the spine. No rubbing of body. Provides extreme and lasting contraction of pelvic blood vessels.

NEUTRAL SITZ BATH

Temperature: 92°F (33.3°C) to 97°F (36.1°C). Foot bath: 102°F (38.9°C) to 106°F (41.1°C). Length of time: 20 minutes to 1 to 2 hours. Apply cold compress to head. Sedative effect.

> Sitz baths are merely as a relaxation for the lumbar, or the lower loco-
> motory area, and should be taken whenever adjustments are to be at-
> tempted . . . this relaxes the system so that the adjustments and the
> muscular movements, where there are alignments that are out of line,
> will be the easier and more active or applicable to the needs of the
> body.   5609-2

VERY HOT SITZ BATH

Temperature: Begin at about 100°F (37.8°C), increase rapidly to 106°F (41.1°C) to 115°F (46.1°C). Foot bath: 110°F (43.3°C) to 120°F (48.9°C). Length of time: 3 to 8 minutes. Apply cold compress to head and neck. At the end, cool the bath to neutral for 1 to 3 minutes. If sweating has occurred, pour cold water over shoulders and chest. Relieves pelvic pain and dysmenorrhea.

REVULSION SITZ BATH

Temperature (same as "Very Hot Sitz Bath"): Begin at 100°F (37.8°C), increase rapidly to 106°F (41.1°C) to 115°F (46.1°C). Foot bath: 110°F (43.3°C) to 120°F (48.9°C). Length of time: 3 to 8 minutes. Apply cold compress to head and neck. At the end, pour pail of cold water onto hips—temperature of water: 55°F (12.7°C) to 65°F (18.3°C). Stimulates deep and superficial blood vessels. Helpful for chronic pelvic inflammatory conditions.

ALTERNATE HOT AND COLD SITZ BATH

Two sitz tubs needed. One tub—temperature: 106°F (41.1°C) to 115°F (46.1°C). Second tub—temperature: 55°F (12.7°C) to 85°F (29.4°C). Foot bath: 105°F (40.5°C) to 115°F (46.1°C). Apply cold compress to head and neck. Length of time: hot water—2 to 3 minutes; then cold—15 to 20 seconds. Return to hot water. Make three complete changes from hot to cold. Provides powerful fluxion (flowing) effects in the pelvic viscera. Helpful for chronic pelvic inflammatory conditions.

Individual Cayce readings do not give such detailed instructions, but these guidelines from Dr. Reilly were submitted as assistance to those whose treatments suggested a sitz bath. Following is a summary of his instruction from *The Edgar Cayce Handbook for Health Through Drugless Therapy*:

For application of a cold, hot, or neutral sitz bath, fill the tub with six to nine inches of water at the recommended temperature; when you are seated in the bath, the water should reach your navel. Place a plastic step stool or foot-rest at the end of the tub to elevate your feet so that your feet will be out of the water and the reaction of the sitz bath can focus on your pelvic area. (Note that this is different from what Dr. Reilly did in his professional practice: placing the feet out of the water rather than *in* a basin of water. Here he is adapting his method.)

Cover the shoulders and upper body with a large towel or blanket. If taking a warm or hot sitz bath, have a cold compress handy to apply to the neck and forehead. Remain in the tub for the recommended length of time, if possible, or take it slowly and gradually work up to the appropriate time limit (maybe after several uses).

Be careful stepping in and out of the tub. Do it cautiously and take your time in order to prevent slipping. Dry off slowly, cover yourself with a large towel or robe, and, if it is bedtime, go to sleep. Or rest at least thirty minutes and then continue with the rest of your day.

DIRECTIONS FROM THE READINGS

For a fifty-three-year-old woman suffering from pruritus, a severe itching of the skin (reading given on October 1, 1942):

> At regular periods—at least once or twice a week—we would take the sitz baths; and this would be, of course, with quite warm water and then quite cold water—and these changed; or sitting in this for at least ten to fifteen minutes each—the hot water, then the cold water, see?
>
> 2470-3

For a forty-three-year-old woman who had experienced a false pregnancy and menopausal symptoms (reading given on April 20, 1931):

> In those periods when there is distress in the pelvic region, these hot and cold flushes, cold feet, general irritation—we would take Epsom Salts sitz baths, see? Prepare at least a small basin or a large washing tub, or such, that the body may sit in same—as hot as the body can bear same—see? and sit until the water is cool, or cold. Then take a thorough *rubdown,* especially enlivening all of the centers along the cerebro-spinal system . . .   4280-9

A thirty-nine-year-old woman had headaches [" . . . cause unknown to doctors . . . " (2602-2, Report #8)] and suffered also from menopausal symptoms (reading given on June 21, 1942):

> Occasionally, outside of the osteopathic adjustments, we would have a good, thorough hydrotherapy treatment. This would include a very light sweat—either the dry or fume type, or the sitz bath. Sitz baths will be well for the body, if these are taken, of course, at the correct period for the body; not just before nor just after the menstrual flow, to be sure . . .   2602-2

TESTIMONIALS/RESULTS

Only a few notations and letters refer to the sitz baths. Several people did not know what they were or how to take them; other references merely noted them as part of a recommended regimen. Edgar Cayce in several letters to readings' recipients would suggest remedies that fit the health problems that they were experiencing. On December 16, 1939, Cayce wrote to Mrs. [1829], a forty–two–year–old woman who had received her second reading earlier that year in April. In a previous letter she described her physical condition, and Cayce responded:

> " . . . I believe if you would take Epsom salts sitz bath for that condition
> {*swollen rectum*} you would get real relief; take them just as hot as
> you can stand them. Then of course change to tap water temperature
> or colder—stay in the Epsom salts bath for 20 minutes or even more,
> put a pound or more of the salts to say five gallons of water. You can
> take this in regular bath tub or even possibly better in a regular
> tub . . . "   1829-2, Report #8

No mention is made of her following this suggestion in a follow–up letter sent nearly five years later, by which time Cayce was ill and no longer giving readings.

A letter mailed to Hugh Lynn Cayce on October 3, 1968, from Robert M. Corey contained this introduction by Gladys Davis: "Here is a letter from someone . . . who did benefit from the treatment for prostatitis." An excerpt from that letter follows:

> " . . . The following is a progress report of the remarkable, lasting results
> of the treatments with Dr. Reilly . . . he set up a schedule of therapeutic
> exercises for me . . . A series of colonic irrigations was started almost
> immediately as were cold sitz baths at bedtime. Changes in diet were
> suggested by Dr. Reilly . . . precise recipes for food preparation accord-
> ing to the Cayce readings . . . About one month after starting treatments
> of every two weeks, there was enough improvement in the prostatitis to
> stop the antibiotic drugs. They have never been taken since . . .

"In conclusion, although not being completely free of the original symptoms all the time, my overall general health has dramatically changed for the better without the use of any antibiotic drugs, and has been maintained by the program set up by Dr. Reilly through guidance of the readings . . . "   3559-1, Report #1

ADDITIONAL INFORMATION

Mentioned in the previous section were some individuals' misunderstandings over just what was a sitz bath. Two rather humorous excerpts reflect this confusion. The first involves a question–and–answer exchange from a twenty–two–year–old woman:

(Q) Please describe Sitz bath prescribed in my reading.
(A) Use a tub and sit down in the water!   578-4

In another reading given to a seventeen–year–old girl on July 30, 1941, this question was asked: "Is it still necessary to take sitz baths?" The answer came: "Not necessary! We just suggested them for the good of the body! If you don't want to take them, don't do it—but they would be well for the body!" (308-8)

Later [308]'s mother explained:

" . . . I hadn't given her the sitz baths because I really didn't know what a sitz bath was. It didn't sound terribly important, but just in case I didn't have this figured out right, I thought we'd better ask about it. Thus the snappy answer . . . "   308-7, Report #4

Dr. Reilly, writing in *The Edgar Cayce Handbook for Health Through Drugless Therapy,* considered the sitz bath "one of the most rewarding uses of water—one that is well worth the trouble. It speeds up circulation and relieves congestion of the glands and the organs of the lower abdomen. It is one of the best methods of invigorating the sex organs and extending their life, especially for men. The cold sitz bath also counteracts fatigue and stimulates elimination." (pp. 206–207) Added benefits include relieving headaches and, if taken just prior to bedtime, assuring a good night's sleep.

Steam/Fume Bath

One of the oldest types for purifying and cleansing skin and body is the steam or fume bath ("steam," if water alone is used in the container, and "fume," if a substance or an oil is added to the boiling water). Highly recommended in the Cayce readings, this method is addressed by various names: steam bath, steam cabinet, sweat bath, cabinet bath, fume bath, vapor cabinet, fume bath cabinet, and Turkish bath. Though available in some form in most health spas today, steam baths can also be rigged up in one's home for personal use. An added benefit is that the head is not enclosed with the steam. The heat becomes more tolerable by exposing the head to room temperature and to oxygen. Having the head exposed, which facilitates the application of cold compresses, is especially important for those individuals who find it difficult to endure heat.

INDICATIONS
Adhesions, arthritis, cataracts, colds, congestion, detoxification, exhaustion, fullness in throat and head, injuries, insomnia, lacerations, lesions, need for relaxation, neuritis, painful areas, pelvic disorders, pleurisy, poor eliminations, skin conditions, sore muscles, toxemia

CONTRAINDICATIONS

High blood pressure, unless controlled by medication; heart and kidney problems; use of illegal drugs; alcohol use; phlebitis; acute skin rashes (such as poison ivy), but psoriasis and eczema are excluded; pregnancy; fever; burns; early menses with cramps, but late menses is OK; use caution with very elderly or feeble individuals; do not get overheated

MATERIALS NEEDED

Access to a health spa facility with steam cabinet or sauna

(For home use) Shower curtain, blankets, or camping tarp—to wrap around you to contain the steam

Wooden stool or chair—to sit upon

Hot plate—place underneath chair or stool or nearby, under covering

Pan of water (open container), coffee pot, tea pot, or vaporizer—to create steam (glass or ceramic pot for certain additives such as Atomidine, rather than metal or plastic)

Towels—to drape over stool, place on floor, set around the neck, and use afterward for shower

Cold compresses (two washcloths dipped in ice water in pan, bowl, or bucket)—to place on forehead and back of neck

Cup of water with flexible straw—to sip while in cabinet

Shower—available to rinse or wash off afterward

FREQUENCY OF APPLICATION

Daily " . . . if there is the strength . . . " (1478-1); every other day; 1, 2, or 3 times a week; every week for 1 month; every 10 days; 4 in 2 weeks; once a week, then twice in 10 days, rest a month before taking another series; once or twice a month; occasionally

AMOUNT OF DOSAGE

(Ratio of water to additive) *One pint of water:* ½ teaspoon of the additive, such as oil of wintergreen; ½ teaspoon witch hazel plus 1 teaspoon balsam of Tolu in solution; 1 or 2 teaspoons or 2 tablespoons, or 1 or 2 ounces of witch hazel; ¾ teaspoon or 1 teaspoon or 1 tablespoon, or 15

or 40 drops of Atomidine; 1 teaspoon witch hazel and 1 teaspoon peanut oil or oil of pine needles; ½ teaspoon oil of wintergreen; ½ teaspoon
sweet oil (olive oil) and 1 teaspoon witch hazel; *½ pint water:* 3 drops
each of Atomidine and wintergreen; 1 teaspoon tincture of iodine; 1
tablespoon spirits of camphor or Atomidine; 1 tablespoon tincture of
iodine (first week) and 1 tablespoon oil of wintergreen (next week); *½ to
1 pint water:* a few drops Atomidine; *1 or 1½ pints water:* 1 or 2 teaspoons
witch hazel; *1½ pints water:* 1 tablespoon wintergreen (first week), 1 tablespoon Atomidine (second week); *2 ounces water:* 2 teaspoons witch hazel;
3 ounces water: 1 teaspoon witch hazel; ½ teaspoon Atomidine; *4 ounces
water:* 1 ounce witch hazel; *6 ounces water:* 1 teaspoon Atomidine; *8 ounces
water:* ¼ ounce Atomidine (use for 5 or 6 steams); *1 quart water:* 1 ounce or
½ teaspoon or 2 teaspoons witch hazel; ½ teaspoon Atomidine; *10 parts
water:* 1 part witch hazel; 1 tablespoon spirits of camphor and olive oil
(equal portions); *1½ gallons water:* ½ pound Epsom salts (saturated solution)—only two readings, 74-1 and 1619-1, mention this additive

ADDITIVES RECOMMENDED

(Equal portions) *1 teaspoon each in 1 pint water:* oil of wintergreen and
tincture of benzoin; witch hazel and rose water; witch hazel and oil of
pine needles; witch hazel and peanut oil; oil of wintergreen and camphor; tincture of balsam (or balsam in essence or solution) and witch hazel

(Equal portions; amounts not specified) pine oil and tolu in solution;
oil of wintergreen and oil of pine; pine oil, witch hazel, and wintergreen; witch hazel and oil of sassafras root or camphor

(Used singly) Aloes, alum, Atomidine, balm of Gilead, Epsom salts,
eucalyptus, iodine, myrrh, oil of lavender, oil of pine needles, oil of
wintergreen, pine oil, sassafras, witch hazel

WHEN TO TAKE THE STEAM/FUME BATH

Before a massage, 1½ hours after eating, after a colonic, in the evening
before retiring, during the period of using the Wet–Cell Appliance, following a series of Atomidine or osteopathic treatments, same day as
osteopathic treatments

LENGTH OF TIME OF APPLICATION

Two to 3 weeks, 1 month (once a week), 8 to 10 treatments
(Remain in cabinet) 1 to 2 minutes at first, increasing time limit gradually; 5 to 8 minutes; 5 to 10 to 15 minutes; 10 to 30 minutes; not longer than 20 minutes; 20 to 25 to 30 minutes; until water boils out

EXPECTED EFFECTS/PURPOSES

Cleanses the organs of elimination: skin, lungs, kidneys
Maintains health and prevents illness
Raises temperature of superficial circulation
Relaxes the body
Helps to eliminate poisons through the respiratory system
Coordinates superficial and deeper circulation

DIRECTIONS

Gyms, recreation centers, or health spas may provide some type of heating equipment to facilitate having a steam or fume bath. If you wish to avoid the cost of membership fees to use these facilities, instructions are also given to construct such a cabinet for home use. Two examples follow—one in a letter from Edgar Cayce and the other from Gladys Davis appended to a reading:

On January 31, 1944, Cayce answered a letter from Mrs. [2602], the wife of [3902], a forty–year–old gentleman who had received a reading. She explained that there was no place in their area, a town in Connecticut, to get steam baths, so Cayce responded:

> " . . . why not make the cabinet to take these in? I am sure [. . .] could do this. You could make it out of oil cloth or canvas ducking. You fasten three sides together; leave one end on the other side open; cut a place in top so head will fit it; then you use like an electric plate to make the steam bath. It doesn't cost very much to do this, and it will be good for everyone of the family . . . "   3902-1, Report #3

Gladys Davis's note, written on December 11, 1937, gave this description:

"A satisfactory Fume Bath may be had by using a huge rubberoid or oilcloth gown fastened around the neck and hanging loosely to the floor, while the body sits on a stool—with only the outside of the gown. In a pint of water boiling on an electric plate or Sterno heat, or the like, under the stool, put half a teaspoonful of the Spirits of Camphor and half a teaspoonful of the Oil of Wintergreen. Sit with these fumes settling over the body for five, ten to fifteen minutes, or until the water has boiled out. Then sponge off the body and have a thorough rubdown ... then an alcohol rub to close the pores of the skin."

Supplement to reading 1455-2

At the A.R.E. headquarters in Virginia Beach are several handmade wooden cabinets with adjustable wooden seats. A deep fryer is situated under the seat with its controls placed through a small opening to the outside for easy access. Towels drape the inside of the cabinet for comfort and protection from excessive heat. The client chooses an additive, a few drops of which are placed in a Pyrex custard cup and floated on top of the boiling water in the container. Then the client steps into the preheated cabinet, sits down, and the wooden doors are closed. The client's head sticks out through a rounded opening at the top, and a towel is draped around the client's neck to prevent the steam from escaping. The pulse in the neck is checked and then rechecked three to five minutes later to monitor any increase. If the second pulse rate is more than thirty beats above the resting pulse, the client needs to discontinue the steam, as this is too rapid an increase and hints of some disturbance or distress in the body. Otherwise, the client remains seated, has sips of water from time to time, and, when sweating occurs, gets cold compresses on the forehead and back of the neck. These compresses enable the client to endure the heat more easily. The compresses may also prevent headaches resulting from dilated blood vessels.

The client chooses to discontinue the steam bath when he or she has worked up a good sweat—one with perspiration running down the body for several minutes. To avoid overheating or dehydration, a time limit of twenty minutes is set, after which the client leaves the cabinet and steps into a tepid shower already turned on by the therapist (*see also* the

chapter on "Showers"). Soap is offered or clients may simply rinse off.
After drying themselves and putting on a robe and slippers, they return
to the dressing room for their massage.

DIRECTIONS FROM THE READINGS

For a fifty-one-year-old woman with acidity as well as problems with
hypertension and lesions (reading given on July 16, 1942):

> Following the colonic, there should be a very mild sweat in the dry
> cabinet—just sufficient to raise the temperature to a sweat. As the
> body begins to perspire (and do keep cold packs on the head, even
> when the fume bath is given—and watch the pulse with this)—put at
> least two teaspoonsful of the Witchhazel in the pint of boiling water for
> the fume bath, so that the steam—as in a croup cup or an open con-
> tainer—settles over the body.   2782-1

For a fifty-one-year-old woman with menopausal complaints who
was also suffering with neuritis (reading given on November 5, 1937):

> Here again {*daughter had just had reading preceding this one; mother
> and daughter were both present for this reading*} we find one of the very
> *best* applications for this body would be the use of the sweat cabinets,
> or fume baths; but alter these for this body. One week use the Tincture
> of Iodine, the next week the Oil of Wintergreen—a tablespoon to half a
> pint of water, and let this boil out—or let just the fumes settle over the
> whole of the body. These will be much preferable to going even to a
> Turkish Bath, or masseurs; but have these done properly for self. Have
> a rubdown afterwards, of course, with massage, and an alcohol rub
> after same—of course—always.
>
>   And these kept up, with the corrections occasionally osteopathically,
> we will find we will renew a body here almost!
>
>   Ready for questions.
>
> (Q) Should this [steam additive] be rubbed into the body?
>
> (A) Rather it would be rubbed *off* of the body! You see, the fumes arise
> from the properties being put in the water that will be heated or boiled,

and the steam settles over the body. It causes a perspiration. You see, the change being wrought is to the respiratory or perspiratory and respiratory system. The fume baths taken in this manner *do not* affect the deeper circulation, but are to the superficial circulation, see? and it aids in removing these drosses; while the very massage of the body, with the drosses out, aids in keeping the body nearer physically fit.

These may be kept as indicated, once a week, twice a month or the like; left off for periods and begun again—and are good for *everyone,* but *particularly* for this body.

(Q) How long should the body stay in the fume bath?

(A) As just given, put a tablespoonful of the properties to half a pint of water and let that *boil out!*

Whether it takes ten minutes, twenty minutes or thirty minutes depends on how hot the bath is and how long it takes the water to boil out.   601-22

A forty-year-old man with poor assimilations was having difficulty relaxing (reading given on December 29, 1941):

Occasionally have not only an exercise that tires the muscles but a perfect relaxation, as with the hydrotherapy treatments—not merely a steam bath but a fume bath, with witchhazel as the fumes, and the rubdown with oils that may be assimilated for stimulating disturbances to the superficial circulation. In the fume bath use a little dry heat, but *more* the fume from witchhazel in water that may settle over the body in the cabinet, see? The proportions would be an ounce of the witchhazel to four ounces of water in a croup cup or the like, or in an open container in the closed cabinet. These will aid the body. Have these with the rubdowns at least once each week. Then have the rubdown with Peanut Oil—if the body would never have arthritis or neuritic reactions.   826-14

For a forty-two-year-old woman with incoordination of circulation and aphonia (loss of voice) tendencies (reading given on September 28, 1937):

(Q) How is a Fume Bath taken?

(A) Either in a Cabinet or in a Gown with the Oil Fumes being about the body; that is, the oilcloth gown, so that the fumes settle over the body. The Oil Solution, of course, would be put in the water that steams under the body.

(Q) How long should one stay in a Fume Bath?

(A) ... If the electrical appliance is used and the fume bath over same, for five to eight minutes.   1079-3

TESTIMONIALS/RESULTS

Mrs. [601], who along with her daughter [480] had been present for the reading (see excerpt under *Directions from the Readings*), wrote on November 16, 1937, eleven days after her twenty–second reading was given:

> "[480] called William M. Berg (Ph.T.) about the cabinet gown before we left N.Y. and he asked $15 for one. After we came home I made one out of oiled silk and used it with an electric vaporizer. It served the purpose and {I} enjoyed an iodine fume bath last Saturday. [480] also had hers and we had a masseur to give us the rubdown after that. I will be able to take another one this Saturday and will leave off while we are away. I have also been using the Atomidine as suggested and feel much more comfortable.
>
> "I am very thankful for what the readings have done for me physically and mentally, even though I do meet with ridicule and lack of understanding. That doesn't bother me in the least for I know I am 'keeping the Way' and learning the meaning of peace and harmony within ... "   601-22, Report #1

Mrs. [2970] was forty–nine years old when she received her second and final reading from Cayce on June 2, 1944. On July 1, 1945, she sent in a letter reporting on her readings. In part her letter stated:

> " ... For the Witch-hazel vapor baths, which were recommended, I did not find any place where they would give this, or in fact knew what it

was. So I found a vaporizer which is used for treating coup, etc., a little electric gadget which will make steam out of water and whatever other liquid is put into it. The tent I made by hanging a sheet up over a line. This made low enough that I could sit on an ordinary kitchen chair, which would not be harmed by the steam bath along with me. The opening in the tent allowed me to leave my head outside and read a book, which I managed to rig up a-la-Rube-Goldberg {*cartoonist, author, and inventor, lived from 1883 to 1970; his name is associated with accomplishing simple tasks through complex means*}. Of course, I did put the little electric steamer under the tent along with me and the chair. I used a mixture of half and half witch-hazel and water.

Altogether the results have been very good . . . my arms are entirely free from the soreness {*she had arthritis tendencies*}, and no soreness in knee joints. Since I started this treatment, and after the 12 or 15 osteopathic treatments, I have done the rest for myself . . . "

2970-2, Report #6

ADDITIONAL INFORMATION

We often forget that the skin is an organ of elimination along with the lungs, kidneys, and colon. It is also our largest organ. In *The Edgar Cayce Handbook for Health Through Drugless Therapy*, Dr. Harold Reilly offers a good explanation of its function:

> "Elimination through the skin is very important, for the skin normally does about one-twentieth of the work of the kidneys. When the skin elimination is speeded up, it can take care of practically one-tenth of the work that the kidneys usually do for the body. Therefore, stimulation through the skin is important for elimination, for it can help kidney function and prevent kidneys from becoming overloaded. Fume baths are useful not only for the skin but also are used for inhalations, thus aiding elimination through the lungs."   (p. 30)

Occasionally clients, especially those who are more used to taking saunas or being in steam rooms, want to place their heads down into the cabinet. Cayce advised against this. Here is one such excerpt:

(Q) Should head be included in the Cabinet recommended?

(A) The head should *not* be in the Cabinet.

If there are periods when those things given to be used *do not* in their activity eliminate the head condition, or because of cold or congestion the head becomes clogged, then we would use an inhalant which we will give here. But if the Fume Baths are taken and the massage between the shoulders and the neck, and the rubdowns, with those properties used as indicated, these should prevent the body from taking cold; of course, with the equalization of the system established.

But if there are the periods of reaction, which may occur—by the body getting the feet wet, or the body remaining in a draft, or leaving the head uncovered too much—we would use an inhalant . . . 1472-2

What about inhaling the steam itself? A few readings advise individuals to stay away from steam rooms, while several others recommended their use, including inhaling the steam. Here is one interesting comment, though, against it: " . . . When around steam, have as much air as is possible. It is well for the lungs, of course, to keep moist—but *not* that *character* of moisture." (1548-3) Perhaps when one takes a sauna or a steam bath (the word *sauna* is not mentioned in the readings), toxins are released into the atmosphere of the enclosure, making it somewhat unhealthy to breathe in.

At the A.R.E. Spa if a client wishes to have more of an inhalant, a few drops of an additive (for example, eucalyptus) may be placed on a tissue on the neck towel directly under the client's nose. Then he or she can easily inhale the aroma as the steam rises from the bottom of the cabinet through the towel. If a client wishes to have the face steamed as well, the neck towel may be opened slightly so that the steam rises through the opening and reaches the face without putting the head into the cabinet.

Obtaining a steam or fume bath, whether at home or in a spa facility, can be an important component of one's cleansing routine.

Turpentine Stupe

A stupe is a cloth wrung out of hot water that usually contains an added medicament for relieving pain or acting as an irritant to stimulate local circulation; it has also been described as medicated water. The cloth is applied externally, supplying moist warmth to sores, lesions, or inflamed areas. In the case of a turpentine stupe, a small amount of spirits of turpentine is added to the hot water into which a cloth or hand towel is dipped, wrung out, and then placed over the bladder or kidney area.

Turpentine in the readings is also used as an ingredient for tonics, inhalants, expectorants, capsules, and resin pellets taken orally. Additionally, turpentine is combined with mutton tallow and spirits of camphor for use in a massage formula. Over seven hundred readings mention turpentine and related substances.

INDICATIONS

(Stupe) Bladder infection, cystitis, kidney infection, kidney stones, painful menstruation, poor eyesight, renal calculus, vaginal pains

(Tonic) Digestion problems, poor eliminations

(Inhalant) Respiratory problems

(Massage formula) Backache, callus (on foot), cold, congestion
(Pellet) Bladder stricture, eliminations
(Expectorant) Excessive mucus

CONTRAINDICATIONS

Some individuals may experience skin sensitivity to the turpentine, causing the nerves in the skin to tingle; though not harmful, it could be unpleasant, so remove the pack after 10 minutes; burning of the skin can also occur, so if the first signs of irritation are felt, remove the pack immediately and wash off the area with plain water

MATERIALS NEEDED

Bottle of spirits of turpentine
Cotton flannel cloth or small hand towel—large enough to cover area of application (kidney or bladder)
One quart jar (four cups) of extremely hot water
One teaspoon—to measure the turpentine
Hot water bottle or electric heating pad—to maintain heat (optional)
Plastic wrap or garbage bag—to protect wet towel from heating pad
Large towel or plastic wrap—to lie on to protect the sheets (optional)

FREQUENCY OF APPLICATION

(Stupe) Depends upon severity of condition, 3 or 4 times throughout the day for pain relief, once or twice a week
(Inhalant) Several times a day
(Massage formula) Each evening
(Capsule) One a day for 3 days, then skip 1 or 2 days
(Tonic) Two or 3 times a day

AMOUNT OF DOSAGE

(Stupe) *Ratio of turpentine to water*—5 drops turpentine: 1 quart warm water; 15 to 20 drops turpentine: 1 quart water; 1 teaspoon turpentine: 1 or 2 ounces or 3 to 4 ounces hot water; 1 teaspoon turpentine: 1 quart boiling water; 1 tablespoon turpentine: 1 quart hot or warm water; 2 tablespoons turpentine: 1 gallon water (weak solution); ½ pint turpentine: 1 to 1½ quarts very hot water

(Pellet) Hold in the mouth a piece of resin about the size of a pea; let it dissolve or chew it—but do not swallow the resin

(Massage formula) Only what the body can absorb

(Tonic) Half a teaspoon

WHEN TO TAKE THE TURPENTINE STUPE

"When there is pain . . . " (243–35); if condition is not too severe, leave pack on for 10 minutes, then remove towel and dry the area

LENGTH OF TIME OF APPLICATION

Ten to 30 minutes (depending upon severity of condition); 1 hour; if pain and discomfort are present, leave pack on until relief is obtained

LOCATION OF APPLICATION

Over the bladder and/or pubic center (on abdomen below navel); over the kidney area (small of lower back/lumbar area); " . . . over the area lower down in the frontal portion . . . " (1112–7)

SIZE OF PACK

Large enough to cover affected area; cotton flannel cloth—4, 5, or 6 thicknesses—or small hand towel; not necessary to apply heat

EXPECTED EFFECTS/PURPOSES

Disintegrates kidney stones (stupe)

Eases pain of urination (stupe)

Activates the digestive organs (tonic)

Acts as a diuretic (inhalant)

Relieves inflammation in trachea and bronchial areas (inhalant)

Prevents infection that may arise in system (inhalant)

Increases eliminations in the kidneys (expectorant)

DIRECTIONS

One of the simplest of the Cayce home remedies, a turpentine stupe (sometimes referred to as a pack) calls for one teaspoon of spirits of turpentine to be placed in one quart (four cups) of very hot water (see *Amount of Dosage* for other ratios). Dip a cloth or small hand towel into the hot water and wring it out. (You may also want to put some plastic wrap or towels on the bed to protect your sheets.) The wet towel should be the size to cover the kidney (lower back) or bladder area (lower abdomen). Place the hot, moist towel directly on the skin, first rotating the cloth back and forth slowly to acclimate the skin before placing it completely on the skin. Leave it on from ten to thirty minutes or longer, depending upon how severe the condition is. It is not necessary to apply heat but, if desired, use a hot water bottle or electric heating pad to maintain the heat, placing a plastic wrap or dry towel between the stupe and the pad.

If the condition is not too severe, apply the pack for ten minutes, remove the towel, and then dry the area with a cloth or towel.

In conjunction with the stupes, your regimen should also include drinking six to eight glasses of water daily plus two to three cups of mild watermelon seed tea per week. Eat an alkaline diet and cut down your intake of white sugar and white flour. This remedy also helps to improve or retain eyesight.

DIRECTIONS FROM THE READINGS

For a four-year-old boy with breathing and circulation problems, cold, and congestion (reading given on May 10, 1944):

> . . . stupes of Turpentine applied over the kidney area would soon release the activity for the kidneys and then just keep the body quiet and give nourishment. These would offer the best that may be given the body . . .
> (Q) Should the Turpentine be diluted to use with stupes?
> (A) Stupes are just a small quantity poured in hot water and rags wrung out of this; about a quart of water. Put about fifteen to twenty drops of Turpentine in the water.   2299-14

For a twenty-four-year-old female dance instructor with toxemia, cholecystitis, and kidney stones (reading given on May 20, 1944):

As we find, from those subluxations that exist between the 7th and 8th dorsal, there has been a hindrance in the amount of nerve energies going to activities between the liver and kidneys. There are those disorders in the gall duct area, the reactions cause heavier flow of activity to be performed by the kidneys in eliminating poisons; that is, lacking in the necessary flow produced accumulations.

These should be tested by x-ray, but if these applications are made we will find we can eliminate this disorder.

About twice each week, Tuesdays and Fridays, when the body is ready to retire, put about 5 drops of Spirits of Turpentine in one quart of warm, little better than lukewarm water, wring a rag or cloth out in same, and place this over the kidney area and let this remain on the back for at least one hour, then remove. Do this for about three times. Then begin (not before) with osteopathic adjustments with special reference to the dorsal, from the 9th dorsal up to the 1st cervical. And while these are being made, during at least twelve to fourteen of such adjustments, do keep having twice a week the stupes of Turpentine over the area. If it causes anxiety in the bladder, do put the same type of Turpentine stupes over the lower portion of the abdomen, to the pubic center, across this whole area, but especially right in the center to the pubic center. These can be kept on or off in regular periods, or irregular periods, depending upon the pain.

With the corrections, do have at least one scientifically given colonic irrigation.   5137-1

TESTIMONIALS/RESULTS

Fifty–five–year–old A.R.E. member, Mrs. Betty L. Walker, from Lincoln Park, Michigan, reported her experiences on August 7, 1980. She had had one gall stone removed in 1968, but in November of 1979 was hospitalized after a kidney stone attack:

" . . . They found a small stone was lodged in the urethra tube. The procedure was to enter the tube with a basket and hope that they could remove it without external surgery. That was not possible. I was told that I would have to drink lots of water and hope that it would be flushed out. That did not happen either so I was sent home . . .

"I used the turpentine packs about three times the first week, {*then*} each week for the next few weeks . . . the doctor x-rayed me to see where the stone was and I told him I think it had moved. This stone did not cause the stabbing-type pains, but it did cause pains of extreme pressure type. The x-ray taken in January showed that the stone had indeed moved down.

"I continued with turpentine packs during the next weeks and was x-rayed again in February. There had been no pain, but the stone was still there. After that I didn't use the packs. The old story of no pain, so I forgot about it. The doctor asked me to get another x-ray in May to check on the case, and there was no sign of it on the print. At no time did I experience any pain like that expected in passing a stone. I would like to assume that the turpentine did indeed dissolve the stone and pass it without even knowing it passed.

"The packs were supposed to be placed on the stomach over the area of the urethra tube, but I am extremely obese and I used it on the reverse side. I surmised that the area rather than the side, back, or front would be the most important, and I would say that it worked.

"I hope that this will encourage any one with kidney stones because the experience of an attack is worse than childbirth. It is necessary that the person be careful not to burn themselves by leaving the pack on too long. I used an aloe cream (any lotion should do) after each pack. I used the half cup turpentine to a quart of warm water, which I saturated a towel and placed over the area mentioned above.

"All I can say is, 'Bless Mr. Cayce, again!'" . . . 1472-16, Report #14

Another A.R.E. member, W.E. Callahan, jotted down on August 1, 1973, the main steps to report success in using the turpentine packs:

"1. Kidney stones (1) diagnosed July 16; 2. Sent for Circulating File July 17; 3. File received July 28 after four additional attacks (mild); 4. First turpentine pack applied July 30 (4 p.m.). Had 1 oz. watermelon {*seed*} tea. Went into labor 10 p.m. July 30. Continuous to 7 a.m. July 31 at which stone passed into bladder. Caught stone 6:50 p.m. July 31, carried to doctor 8/1/73. Many thanks. Stomach burned from turpentine, but will be O.K. {*in a*} couple of days!"   1839-1, Report #3

August 10, 1976, brings another account, this one from A.R.E. member M. Saraydarion, who borrowed the Circulating File on Kidney Stones for her husband. She writes:

"I am sorry for keeping {*the file*} so long, but we had difficulty deciphering the best treatment for my husband, and secondly we wanted to wait until we saw some improvement.

"At the time when we received the file, my husband had a continuous dull pain in his right kidney area and sometimes in the groin. This dull ache began after an extremely bad attack, which was diagnosed as a kidney stone by our doctor and a radiologist.

"He got his attack on July 10. On July 31 he began drinking one ounce of watermelon seed tea each day. He also started applying turpentine packs every evening. By August 4 the constant pain was gone. In its place was occasional pain. By August 8, when he stopped the turpentine packs, he no longer had any pain, occasional or otherwise.

"Whether the stone passed intact and he didn't catch it or it dissolved, we don't know. But the point is, he now feels perfectly well and for that we are extremely grateful. We are truly amazed . . . "
                                                                               1839-1, Report #4

ADDITIONAL INFORMATION

Turpentine in large amounts is obtained from several species of pine in the southern United States. Most people are familiar with its potent odor in paints and varnishes, where it is used as a solvent and thinning agent. Due to its antiseptic properties and "clean scent," it is added to many cleaning and sanitary products. Turpentine is also used as a topical antiseptic for rheumatic and neuralgic ailments.

Also called spirits of turpentine, oil of turpentine, wood turpentine, gum turpentine, and turp, this aromatic yellow to brown semifluid comes from the sapwood of pines, firs, and other conifers. It is made up of two principal components: an essential oil and a type of resin (called rosin). The fluid is obtained by the distillation of rosin from the trees. The essential oil (oil of turpentine) can be separated from the rosin by steam distillation; and commercial turpentine, or turps, is this oil of turpentine. When pure, it is a colorless, transparent, oily liquid with a penetrating odor and a characteristic taste. Its vapor can burn the skin and eyes as well as damage the lungs and respiratory and central nervous systems. It is also highly flammable.

Turpentine has been used medically since ancient times as a treatment for lice, in chest rubs, and for intestinal parasites.

Violet Ray Device

One of several electrical appliances recommended in the Cayce readings, the Violet Ray is a unique instrument. During Cayce's day it was available from pharmacies or electrical appliance stores for use by physicians and laypeople. Today, because of its positive effect on the skin, cosmetologists, beauticians, and aestheticians use it for psoriasis, acne, and hair growth.

The Violet Ray is a user–friendly, hand–held device that can be purchased along with a variety of glass applicators such as a bulb, a comb rake, or a rod, each with a specific purpose. The glass applicator is inserted into the tip of the hand–held section. After being plugged in and turned on, the appliance becomes a high–voltage, low–amperage (current) source of static electricity. The discharge creates a violet color (hence, its name), a pleasant ozone smell—and a sizzling noise! It "has an output of about 50,000 volts and a frequency of over one million cycles per second. The current is diffused onto an electrical 'spray' of minute, harmless units" by the glass applicator. (From the *Instruction Manual for Use of the Violet Ray*)

Mentioned in nearly nine hundred readings, the Violet Ray was recommended for a wide variety of conditions, due probably to its three important effects: light, heat, and ozone. (See *Additional Information* for further discussion.)

INDICATIONS

Anxiety, arthritis, baldness, insomnia, cancer (used with carbon or animated ash), cataracts, catarrh, chest pain, circulation problems, cold feet, digestion problems, dry skin, dysmenorrhea, earache, exhaustion, eye problems, eyestrain, fading hair color, goiter tendency, hair disorders, hair growth, headaches, itchy or scaly scalp, nervous system disorders, poor eliminations, reproductive organ disorders, restlessness, rheumatism, Riggs's disease (pyorrhea alveolaris), ringworm, sinus trouble, skin abrasions, swallowing difficulties, uterine fibroid tumor

CONTRAINDICATIONS

Do not use on the same day when: taking Atomidine, receiving spinal adjustments or X–rays, taking medicinal drugs, alcohol, or using other electrical treatments; do not use during the week of doing Kriya yoga

Not mentioned in the readings but considered precautionary measures: do not use or operate if you have a pacemaker; do not use the eye applicator on your eyelids with lens implants or contact lenses

Some individuals were told to set up a better cleansing and elimination process in their systems before using the device; another was told not to use it during hot weather in the summertime (3450-2) or if one has gotten more sunshine than usual (325-58)

Any redness or itching from using the Violet Ray is not harmful

(For further explanation of contraindications see *Additional Information.*)

MATERIALS NEEDED

Violet Ray device—sold with bulb applicator

Various applicators (comb rake, rod, small bulb, etc.)—sold separately (optional)

FREQUENCY OF APPLICATION

Daily, leveling off to several days a week to several times a month; every other evening; once, twice, 3, or 4 times a week; 2 or 3 days, rest 2 or 3 days, use again; occasionally

WHEN TO TAKE THE APPLICATION

Evenings before retiring; when feeling tired or languid; after salt packs—plain or Epsom (apply on same area as packs); after spinal manipulations or massage; after castor oil packs; before or after applying a potato poultice (for the eyes); days when not taking Atomidine (see *Contraindications*); when feeling a " . . . slowing of the pulsations through the lower limbs . . . " (394-9)

LENGTH OF TIME OF APPLICATION

Thirty seconds to several minutes; ½ to ¾ of a minute; 1 to 1½ minutes; 2, 2½, 3 to 5 minutes; not longer than 3 minutes; 5 to 15 minutes; 2 minutes in the beginning, gradually increasing to 15 minutes; 10 days or 2 weeks; 4 to 6 weeks; for eyes—not longer than 1 minute; " . . . until there is the feeling of the whole internal forces being electrified . . . " (264-11)

Note: Avoid overuse; some devices today can overheat, so turn off before reaching 10 minutes and allow for a cooling period—20 minutes—before reusing; other devices can be operated for up to 15 minutes, allowing a cooling period—20 minutes—before reuse

LOCATION OF APPLICATION

Abdomen, across the diaphragm, across the groin, along both sides of the spine (with downward circular motion), armpits, bottoms of feet, chest, directly over closed eyelids, down the limbs, neck, on scalp and around head (comb rake applicator), over the whole circulatory system, palms of hands, shoulders, solar plexus, throat, vaginal area (rod applicator), " . . . where the strains have existed . . . " (4143-1), " . . . apply it *all over* the body, from the tip of the toes to the top of the head . . . " (1091-1)

EXPECTED EFFECTS/PURPOSES

Stimulates superficial circulation

Rejuvenates the nervous system and prevents its " . . . batteries from running down . . . " (2528-4)

Assists with digestion and elimination problems

Promotes relaxation

Stimulates and assists in proper drainage from the system

Helps relieve various reproductive disorders

Has a strengthening effect on the body and on nerve tissue

Cleanses the bloodstream

Stimulates lymphatic and capillary circulation

Reduces glandular swelling

Eases pain

Prevents " . . . adherence of tissue in the organs of the pelvis . . . " (601-17)

Stimulates " . . . coordination between the cerebrospinal and the sympathetic system . . . " (1584-1)

DIRECTIONS

Instructions accompany the appliance when it is purchased. Choose the glass applicator you wish to use and insert it into the opening at the tip of the device with a straight pushing motion, but giving it a slight twist. Hold the applicator by its stem and gently insert, eliminating pressure on its delicate glass structure. After the proper applicator has been inserted, plug the machine into any electrical outlet AC or DC current 110 volts. Place the glass bulb directly on the skin before turning it on from the control knob at the opposite end. This action prevents the mild static electric shock that would otherwise occur.

You may also first test the proper strength of the current by turning the control knob—to the left decreases the current, to the right increases it. When you have decided on the proper strength, turn the knob until the machine is off, place the applicator on the skin, and then turn the knob back to on until you have reached the chosen proper current. Now begin the treatment.

Contact with the skin should be maintained throughout the short session (usually lasting from thirty seconds to several minutes). Do not hold the applicator still—in one place—but move it back and forth across the area to be treated. You may also guide it with your other hand. The skin should be dry and free of oil or any lubricant or lotion (see *Additional Information* for more on this topic).

While giving the treatment, hold the device at the farthest end from the applicator (toward the control knob). If it is held too close to the applicator, the current might jump back, causing a slight shock to the operator. When finished, first turn the machine off at the control knob before removing the device from the body—preventing another possible shock. Lastly, unplug the machine from the outlet.

Because the devices sold today can overheat due to high resistance, turn off the device before ten minutes of use (see *Length of Time of Application*). It is advised that one begin with a short session, gradually increasing the time with each use, if that seems necessary and beneficial.

DIRECTIONS FROM THE READINGS

A seventy–three–year–old woman who received a total of twenty-seven readings was suffering from dementia and incoordination of the nervous system (reading given on April 10, 1940):

> We would use the Hand Violet Ray; this for the nerve forces will aid especially, if it is *gradually* used across the abdominal area; this given just before the body retires, or when it is prepared for rest of evenings, will aid in better rest and will aid in relaxing the body and stimulating better eliminations. Take about fifteen minutes in making the application; not going through it hurriedly, but each portion to which it is applied given due consideration. Use the bulb applicator, so that it may be used as a character of massage; along the spine—but *here, always* downward, *never* the strokes upward! and also across the abdomen, slowly. Though there will be some interference and some resistance to this, at first, we find that it may gradually be used. Across the abdomen it would be rather as a kneading or a massaging. Fifteen minutes in all. And we will find this to be a most helpful portion of the treatments in the present.   1553-20

For a fifty-four-year-old woman suffering from poor circulation, acidity, and spinal subluxations (reading given on April 2, 1938):

(Q) What causes the hair to fade? How may life be restored?
(A) Use the scalp applicator of the violet ray occasionally.
The general stimulation to the activities of the glandular system, with these applications indicated, will aid much. For remember, all of these—the cuticle, the skin, the hair, the activities of all of these natures—arise from the functionings of the thyroid system, see? . . .
                                                                                    1563-1

An adult female with neuritis, toxemia, and poor eliminations (reading given on May 16, 1929):

(Q) Is there anything that can be done for my eyes, so that I won't have to wear glasses?
(A) The correction of the conditions in the cervical, and the treatment with the Violet Ray will materially aid these. Especially will the body use, after the first three to five treatments—or after the 2nd or third week—the Violet Ray applicator for the eyes, but not treating the eyes longer than one minute . . .   5571-1

TESTIMONIALS/RESULTS

A number of people had difficulty either locating the Violet Ray to purchase it or finding a cooperative physician to administer the treatment. Even some doctors familiar with Cayce's work disagreed over the length of the treatment specified in their patient's reading or believed the device was too strong for their patient's use. Several individuals confused it with other devices that were on the market. A postscript from Cayce's secretary, Gladys Davis, in a letter to Mrs. [2843] written on October 5, 1943, gave a brief account of her experience with the device:

" . . . The readings suggested the violet ray for me 20 years ago, and I haven't worn glasses since. So I know from experience what it can do . . . "   2843-4, Report #2

Edgar Cayce himself answered questions and made comments in response to concerns expressed in recipients' letters. Here is one example:

> "... Don't think there is any chance for harming yourself with the use of same [the Violet Ray]. Of course, were you to use the Ultra Violet there would be—but with the Violet Ray—no. Never heard of any one having trouble with such—use only as directed and only as long as suggested. Think you will have no trouble at all ...
>
> "Let me hear from you as to how you come along ... "
>
> 1551-3, Report #2

One female adult, about age seventy, wrote on May 26, 1924, about her experience:

> "... The nerve plexus between shoulders where you said a lesion had formed gave me much pain during the winter. I took a few treatments of the violet ray, the relief was certainly wonderful. Within the next few days I will begin treatment and trust to get it this time in a consecutive way as you prescribed or directed. I feel sure I will be benefited ... "
>
> 232-1, Report #2

In reply to a questionnaire sent out by the A.R.E. Mrs. [3246] wrote this report on February 26, 1952:

> "When I got my physical reading in 1943, I followed Mr. Cayce's advice and had six osteopathic treatments as outlined, followed up the next day with the violet ray vibrator (bulb). The treatments gave me great relief from nervous tension and I still follow this treatment from time to time, when I feel it to be necessary. As for the mental attitude: I have tried to correct this as much as possible. I never suffer from loss of voice since I took the first treatments. I did not consult a physician previous to the treatments. I never had too much faith in physicians ... "
>
> 3246-2, Report #2

Another woman had minimal success in following her protocol. On

March 19, 1951, Mrs. [263] reported:

> "I used the violet ray for a time and it helped me, but at the time I was
> in such a mental and emotional state that I think it took away the help
> I did get from it. It did help quiet my nerves, though. I used it for about
> six months . . . "   263-13, Report #3

On October 30, 1939, Mrs. [808] wrote about her friend [1935], a thirty-
six-year-old woman whom she had recommended for a reading:

> "[1935]'s eye has healed up completely and she has no trouble with it
> at all now. She has been very faithful about the violet ray machine,
> etc., and feels rewarded for her effort. Also wanted me to tell you how
> grateful she is."   1935-1, Report #2

After speaking on the telephone to Mr. [2302]'s daughter who requested another reading for her seventy-year-old father, Gladys Davis
noted on May 12, 1942, that he:

> " . . . has had 43 osteopathic treatments, and is *so much* better in every
> way except his vision. He complained recently of the violet ray stinging
> his eyes when used full strength, so they had to turn it to about a fourth
> of its strength; felt possibly that was a sign of vision being awakened.
> They know he is improved, and want to continue everything if it is
> necessary . . . "   2302-4, Report #2

They wished to get further instructions in the follow-up reading.

A short note provided by Gladys Davis, concerned Mrs. [2790]'s success:

> " With using Violet Ray regularly, the glandular swelling was reduced
> and goitre did not develop."   2790-3, Report #1

The next reading two months later confirmed that the conditions
were much improved.

On February 3, 1952, Mrs. [3386] sent in a report on the follow–up to her previous readings. Included in her account was this information:

> " . . . After the massage and the violet-ray apparatus the insomnia was much improved and in a few weeks I was sleeping like a baby and still am . . . "   3386-2, Report #7

Mrs. [4471] had a total of four readings in 1924. One–and–a–half months after her second reading she wrote to Cayce on May 14, 1924:

> "You have asked that I let you know as to my progress in the treatment as prescribed in the two readings (March 4th and March 31st) given me. Am very sorry that I cannot report favorably. I have taken the osteopathic and the violet ray treatments very faithfully and hopefully—and regret to say that I am no better. My knees creak just as badly and my ears ring just as loudly as when I started. I still have that awful tired and exhausted feeling. Feet and legs in same condition as when I began the treatments.
> "Now, what is wrong—what can you do? Has there been a mistake? Will you make another reading?
> "Please let me hear from you . . . "   4471-2, Report #2

Cayce did give her a check reading in May and another in July, which was very hopeful regarding her improvement. She eventually saw another osteopath who believed that poisons from her tonsils and teeth were causing most of her difficulties, and she concurred with this assessment.

The final testimonial comes from an affidavit filed on January 22, 1921, by Mr. [4959], who received a reading the previous October 1920. A note added in place of the reading states that the reading "is not on file with the Edgar Cayce Foundation or elsewhere according to available records." The affidavit describes abscesses in both ears as a result of getting water in the ears following a swimming vacation in Reading, Pennsylvania. Even after he consulted with two doctors and a specialist,

the abscesses worsened, creating "running ears" and affecting also his
nose and throat:

> " . . . until in the middle of October I could hardly hear and had great
> difficulty in breathing and speaking. I got in touch with Mr. Cayce, and
> he came to Birmingham {*Alabama*} and gave me a reading upon his
> arrival here. Mr. Cayce knew very little of my trouble in my head, but in
> the reading went thoroughly into the trouble, explained where the
> trouble was, and how it could be cured, telling me to stop treatment
> with the ear specialist and take up osteopathy and electric violet ray
> treatment. I have followed his advice as closely as it was possible for
> me, and am still following the treatment, and today my hearing is en-
> tirely restored, my ears have stopped running since the beginning of
> December, and I have again started singing; with the exception of a
> little trouble with my nose (which I know will disappear in time), I am
> perfectly well . . . "   4959-1, Report #1

ADDITIONAL INFORMATION

As noted in the introduction at the beginning of this chapter, three
important effects of the Violet Ray are light, heat, and ozone. Perhaps
because of these effects, the device has a wide variety of application.

Electricity coming from the Violet Ray gives off light, a useful therapy
that was used in earlier times by osteopaths to combat infection (before
the advent of antibiotics). The introduction of light into body tissues
has only recently begun to be scientifically recognized.

Heat, created in the device's generating part, may be only slightly
discernible to the person receiving the treatment. The increase in heat
stimulates superficial circulation (lymphatic and capillary). As a result,
toxins are flushed away and the body's organs are strengthened.

Ozone, a form of oxygen (O_3), is produced from the combination of
static electricity and the oxygen in the air. Found in the atmosphere in
minute quantities, it is the familiar odor detected after a thunderstorm.
In some areas, ozone is utilized as an alternative to chlorine in destroying
bacteria in the water supply. Cayce in several readings encouraged people
to inhale this distinct odor of ozone, stating that it would be beneficial.

An interesting note regarding the Violet Ray is that the coil in this device was invented by renowned genius and electrical scientist, Nikola Tesla (1856–1943). As the voltage, using a transformer, moves through the coil, it is increased, ionizing the gas in the bulb. This ionization produces charged particles that emanate from the bulb's surface. The high frequency and charged particles create a mild heating effect, which increases circulation and dilates the superficial blood vessels wherever the device is applied, thus promoting healing.

Some precautions are advised in the use and application of the Violet Ray, often specific to the particular individual. It would be incorrect to assume that the device is appropriate in every condition for which it was prescribed in Cayce's readings. Its recommendation, in other words, depends upon the cause of a particular condition and not on the diagnosis of a health problem. Some instances of contraindications include the following:

Contrary to some written instructions, no mention is made in the readings of any oil or lubricant that is necessary to be put on the skin prior to using the Violet Ray. The one exception is a reading for an asthmatic, arthritic sixty–three–year–old woman who was treated several years later at the Cayce Hospital. In her second reading the following exchange took place:

(Q) Has the Violet Ray caused any burn?
(A) No. Only the body should not allow same to be used when there's too much moisture, or too long in one place. The body may use talc powder over the portions where the appliance is applied, and we will not have burns.   5556-2

Since sometimes a massage was given just before the Violet Ray, implying that the skin would be moist, Cayce in one instance gave this instruction:

. . . we would massage the body thoroughly with an equal combination of Mutton Suet, Spirits of Turpentine and Spirits of Camphor. Massage what the body will absorb, but do not have the body too damp from the properties when the violet ray (bulb applicator) is applied. Rub off the body rather dry, but let the properties be massaged into the body, or be *in* the skin when the violet ray is applied; for it will drive same more into those areas where there have been the inclination for congestion.

389-10

Another woman, advised to get a fume steam bath, followed by a hot and cold shower, then a massage followed by an alcohol rub, was told: " . . . (after the body is thoroughly dried from the hydrotherapy measures and the masseur's treatment) use the Violet Ray . . . " (1678-1)

A number of other precautionary measures are mentioned throughout the readings, such as not using the Violet Ray on the same day that one is taking Atomidine or " . . . *during* the times {when} the {spinal} adjustments are being taken!" (1584-1) One individual asked if " . . . the yoga practice of Kriya {is} causing any ill effects"; she was told that " . . . this is very well . . . for these exercises have a stimulating effect. However, *do not* use these during the period the Violet Ray is used, for that week!" (813-2)

Medicines and drugs were noted in this excerpt:

> "*Do not take medicinal properties while these [vibrations] are being applied, see?* either the osteopathic forces or the electrical treatments! Take no drugs." 4843-1

Alcohol is also to be avoided. " . . . *Do not* use in the system during the treatments . . . with the Violet Ray—for *these* are detrimental, and would burn tissue, with this in system . . . " (5525-1) Even inhaling the brandy fumes from a charred oak keg might cause irritations to the body if used in conjunction with the Violet Ray.

Some individuals were told not to use the Violet Ray until they had established a better cleansing and elimination process in their systems. One woman was told " . . . not {to} use the Violet Ray through the hot weather." (3450-2) Another reading explained: "When the body gets the sunshine it is not necessary for so much of the violet ray." (325-58) Also,

" . . . if the X-Ray flashes are used we would not use the violet ray . . .
leave off the machine while the X-Ray treatments are being given!"
(325–64)

As mentioned in *Contraindications*, persons with pacemakers should
not operate the device or receive a treatment, and those with lens implants are advised not to use the eye applicator on their eyelids.

In a letter from Cayce on March 24, 1936, to Mrs. [954], a thirty–eight-
year-old woman who needed a bit more instruction on the use of the
Violet Ray, he mentioned a further caution not noted elsewhere:

> " . . . with the rod applicator, you are taking considerable amount of
> electricity, so don't give the treatment too long at a time in the begin-
> ning, and be sure to take off your watch or jewelry or anything of the
> kind when taking a treatment . . . "   954-2, Report #3

In conclusion, here are several excerpts from the readings that further describe the workings of the Violet Ray device:

> . . . the violet ray is only an electrical vibration that coordinates the
> vibratory forces of the bodily functioning itself—which means the cir-
> culation as related to the nerve forces of the body. Then, to revitalize
> the old blood cells without new being builded makes for a deterioration
> quick with same and becomes detrimental rather than helpful.
>
> But to have these to coordinate together, or to have the rebuilding
> and *then* the revitalizing, it is as the addition of strength to the body
> under such conditions.   1187-9

> . . . the Violet Ray. This is a high voltage, stimulating all centers that
> are as the crossroads, the connections between the various portions of
> the physical body functioning, the mental attitudes and attainments,
> as well as the sources of supply . . .   263-13

In Cayce's own reading we have these comments:

> . . . The organs of the whole system need vibrations, either through

deep manipulation or those of the violet ray forces to keep each organ
vibrating to its proper form within the system. Those of the violet ray,
without the amperage, which gives the voltage directly to organs of the
system. We would do that.   294-7

Warm/Hot Water Beverage

People often comment that some of the recommended suggestions from the Cayce readings remind them of ancestral folk remedies, sometimes long forgotten until discovering them in the readings. Such a remedy is the subject of this chapter: drinking a glass of warm or hot water shortly after awakening. At least ten individuals were given this advice.

Treating constipation is one of several conditions noted in the readings for using this remedy.

INDICATIONS

Acidity, constipation, eyestrain, incoordination between elimination and assimilation, nausea, poor digestion

MATERIALS NEEDED

Mug, glass, or cup filled with warm or hot—but not too hot—water; not tepid water

Pinch of table salt (iodized) may be added to the water; or ¼ teaspoon salt in a little warm water (optional)

FREQUENCY OF APPLICATION

Mornings; a few mornings—for settling the stomach; 3 mornings in succession, leave off, then take again if necessary—for eyestrain

AMOUNT OF DOSAGE

One-half to ¾ of a glass, 1 glass, 1½ glasses

WHEN TO TAKE THE DOSAGE

Upon awakening, first thing in the morning, before breakfast

EXPECTED EFFECTS/PURPOSES

Will " . . . clarify the system of poisons . . . " (311-4)

Speeds sluggish digestion

Quenches thirst

Detoxifies and cleanses the body system

Promotes eliminations and " . . . acts on the kidneys themselves . . . " (3798-4)

Helps to throw out from the stomach " . . . those poisons or accumulations by the rest periods . . . " (843-2)

DIRECTIONS

Between the period of waking up and eating breakfast, take a glass, mug, or cup and add warm or hot water—it should not be too tepid. You may get the warm water from the tap, from a coffee machine, or from a stove pan of water heated just prior to the boiling point. The water should be warm but not too hot to drink comfortably. A small amount of table salt may be added to the water—a pinch or one-fourth of a teaspoon. Drink it at a regular pace, without rushing or gulping it down.

DIRECTIONS FROM THE READINGS

A fifty-two-year-old man who felt burning, achy, and tired upon awakening each morning was advised to do some stretching exercises while lying in bed before he consumed his hot water drink (reading given on April 16, 1935):

> . . . Drink a glass of warm water, hot as may be taken, first on awak-
> ening; and this will be helpful to the throwing out and carrying out of
> the stomach those poisons or accumulations by the rest periods, see?
> 843-2

A female adult with poor eliminations and arthritis tendencies asked
a range of health questions (her physical, mental, and spiritual reading
was given on August 7, 1931):

> . . . Drink at least one glass of *warm* water before breakfast. Would be
> well to have a small pinch of salt in same. Iodized salt would be the
> better. In between the breakfast and luncheon there should be at least
> three to four glasses of water, and the same in the afternoon and
> evening.   2843-1

TESTIMONIALS/RESULTS

From the follow-up reports in the Cayce readings, no information
reveals the outcome of following this advice. Accounts from two different sources, however, attest to the usefulness and benefit of the hot
beverage drink. One comes from an email sent on July 17, 2011, to the
author from longtime A.R.E. member Ann Jaffin in Silver Spring, Maryland:

> "Since you wrote a 'True Health' article [column in *Venture Inward
> Newsletter*] about the benefit of drinking hot water the first thing in
> the morning (Summer 2010 issue), I've been doing that with good re-
> sults. The readings say that this practice will flush yesterday's food out
> of the stomach. I'd had some reflux for several months and, since I've
> been drinking the hot water in the morning, the reflux has diminished.
> My doctor has cut my reflux medication in half and I feel better!
> Thanks!"

The second account appeared in "Your Health," a newspaper column
by Dr. Peter Gott in *The Virginian-Pilot* ("The Sunday Break," November 2,
2008, p. 13). A reader of the column had had her gallbladder removed

twenty years ago and suffered from irregular bowel movements afterwards. She remembered an old folk medicine remedy from a book by
Dr. D.C. Jarvis (*Folk Medicine*):

> "The doctor said to simply drink a mug of hot water one-half hour be-
> fore breakfast every day. Figuring it harmless and, at worst, that it
> would fill my bladder a little faster, I tried it. I could immediately feel
> the water emptying my stomach of the contents from the night before.
> Within just a few days, I was completely regulated. It was amazing.
>
> "I told my doctor of this simple remedy, and he said it was one of the
> best. When I asked why no one ever mentions it, he responded that
> most patients and doctors feel that it is too easy. I guess in today's
> society, medication is king."
>
> {*Dr. Gott replied:*} "This is a novel remedy I had nearly forgotten
> about until your letter arrived. The action of the hot water works to
> speed sluggish digestion . . . Perhaps the key is simply the temperature
> of the liquid and the time it is consumed."

The following readings' extract cites the effect of warm water upon
digestion, describing the stomach as a medicine chest for the system:

> . . . Well to drink *always plenty* of water, before meals and after meals—
> for, as has oft been given, when any food value *enters* the stomach
> *immediately* the stomach becomes a storehouse, or a medicine chest
> that may create all the elements necessary for proper digestion within
> the system. If this *first* is acted upon by aqua pura, the reactions are
> more near normal. Well, then, each morning upon first arising, to take
> a half to three-quarters of a glass of *warm* water; not so hot that it is
> objectionable, not so tepid that it makes for sickening but this will
> clarify the system of poisons . . . Occasionally a pinch of salt should be
> added to this draught of water . . .   311-4

ADDITIONAL INFORMATION

The suggestion for an early–morning warm–water drink is scattered
lightly throughout the readings, ranging from readings given in 1910,

through the '30s, and up to 1942. On a few occasions the individual was advised to take this remedy with no definite reason offered. In other readings, the suggestion came in answer to the recipient's question; but in several instances, a specific purpose for the drink was given.

Better known is the Cayce recommendation for many individuals to drink at least six to eight glasses of water daily. This action will help flush the kidneys, ensure proper eliminations, and " . . . build the body to its normal resistance." (583-4) The reading excerpt 2843-1 in *Directions from the Readings* describes how this goal of eight glasses of water a day could be accomplished: " . . . In between the breakfast and luncheon there should be at least three to four glasses of water, and the same in the afternoon and evening."

Wet-Cell Appliance

Sometimes referred to as the Wet–Cell Battery, this device is a form of electrical therapy or electrical medicine in that it produces a small, yet measurable electric current (a DC voltage of about one-fiftieth the output of a common 1.5 volt flashlight battery). According to the Cayce readings, the Wet-Cell Appliance stimulates the growth of nerve tissue by introducing to the body low-frequency and low-amperage wave forms that help create elements or compounds which may be deficient in the body.

Its charge consists of a solution of chemicals, usually made up of distilled water, copper sulfate, sulfuric acid CP, zinc, and willow charcoal. Two poles, one of nickel (negative) and one of copper (positive), extend into the solution contained in a heavy crock. Lead wires are attached to the ends of the poles; one extending to the body of the individual, the other to a solution jar that has a spiral or U–shaped loop immersed in its solution. The ingredient in the solution jar is seemingly transmitted vibrationally to the body, working through the nervous system. Solutions in the jar may include Atomidine, gold chloride, camphor, or silver nitrate. In some cases, this arrangement is more beneficial than taking internally certain minerals such as iodine and gold. Metal disks located on the ends of two wires are placed on the body in specific, designated locations, depending upon the individual's health condition.

The Wet-Cell Appliance is recommended in nearly six hundred Cayce readings for a wide range of health conditions—over 150 different ailments—and is used almost exclusively as a "curative" treatment. During the time of applying the device, one is to rest and relax, pray and meditate, or read selections from the Bible. Because of individuals' differences from reading to reading, it is highly recommended that users of the device study the Circulating File regarding their particular ailments and follow the Wet-Cell directions given in a reading that closely matches their own bodily symptoms. Directions included with the device, a DVD, and booklets containing helpful descriptions and instructions are also available.

It might take a month of use before effects are felt, so application requires persistence and patience. To aid in distributing the energies from this device, manual therapies in the form of massage, osteopathy, and the like are often recommended.

INDICATIONS

Abrasions, adhesions, alcoholism, Alzheimer's disease, amyotrophic lateral sclerosis (Lou Gehrig's disease), arthritis, asthma, brain disorders, burns, cancer, cerebral hemorrhage, cerebral palsy, cirrhosis of the liver, colitis, deafness, debilitation, depression, diabetes, Down's syndrome, epilepsy, eye disorders (blindness, color blindness, glaucoma, iritis), glandular disorders, goiter, hypertension, impaired or atrophied nerve endings, incoordination between sympathetic and cerebrospinal nervous systems, infantile paralysis, insomnia, mental disorders, migraine headaches, multiple sclerosis, muscular atrophy, muscular dystrophy, neurasthenia, neuritis, obesity, paralysis, Parkinson's disease, poor circulation and elimination, prostatitis, Recklinghausen's disease, retardation, rheumatoid arthritis, ringworm, sciatica, scleroderma, senility, skin disorders (dermatitis), spasms, sterility, torticollis, toxemia, tumors (brain, breast, lymph, uterus), ulcers, venereal disease, vertigo, vitiligo

CONTRAINDICATIONS

No alcoholic or intoxicating drinks during the period of using the Wet-Cell; " . . . do not let the body take any element that will even produce an extra amount of alcohol of any character in the system . . . " (2215-1)

MATERIALS NEEDED

Nonbreakable, nonmetal container (to hold 1½ gallons of solution), " . . . but the container would be at least half a gallon larger." (1800-25)— that is, a 2-gallon container

Lid for container made of same material

Distilled water—1½ gallons

Ingredients to be placed in the container (according to a specific reading)

Copper and nickel poles and plates

Connecting wires

Solution jar (with plain lid plus lid with U-shaped or spiral lead loop)

Ingredients for the solution jar (according to a specific reading)

Emery paper (used for polishing the rods and disks)

Mixing stick (to stir contents of the container)

Brush with handle

[Except for distilled water and ingredients for the solution jar, the previous items are included in a starter kit.]

Large plastic chest for storing all the supplies (optional)

FREQUENCY OF APPLICATION

Depends upon one's reason for usage and the information from the Cayce readings, daily

LENGTH OF TIME OF APPLICATION

Depends upon one's reason for usage and the information from the Cayce readings, 30 minutes, for 3 weeks

WHEN TO USE THE WET-CELL APPLIANCE

When one's condition has progressed to a more serious stage, if one's body is seriously deficient in one or more compounds or elements, if the nerve endings are seriously impaired or atrophied

EXPECTED EFFECTS/PURPOSES

Stimulates growth of nerve tissue
Balances the glandular system
Supplies the necessary electrical vibrations needed for healing
Attunes the body's atomic vibrations to normalcy
Helps to activate organs of the body
Stimulates an increase in leucocytes
Equalizes circulation
Relieves liver and gall duct conditions

DIRECTIONS

The following explanation must be very general due to the varia-tions of applications found in the readings as to ingredients of the solu-tions, length of time of application, and placement positions of the metal disks upon the body. As stated earlier, it is highly recommended that you study the readings based on your particular ailment, as found in the Circulating Files, and follow the instructions given that matches closely your condition. Also read and study carefully the instructions accompanying the appliance for assembling the battery and mixing the solutions.

The first step is to set up the nonbreakable two–gallon container. Wash it and dry it thoroughly. Polish the nickel and copper rods, then add the ingredients to the container (in a specific order) and stir the solution with a wooden stick until most of the charcoal is absorbed into the mixture. You may have to attach the copper and nickel rods to the container's lid. Put the lid on top of the container with the rods project-ing down into the solution. For the first session the battery should rest at least twenty–four hours before it is used and should remain in the same place throughout the entire (usual) thirty–day cycle of application.

Like the Radio–Active Appliance, the disks should not come in contact with each other or with other metal objects after they are attached to the appliance. Before and after each use, the face of the disk that touches the skin must be thoroughly cleaned with fine emery paper.

Next, set up the solution jar, whose contents depend upon the reading you are following. The four-ounce jar holds about three ounces of solution. About twenty minutes before your session, screw the jar lid with its lead loop attachment onto the solution jar. Polish the nickel and copper plates, then hook up the wires: Attach the long red wire (with the small copper plate) to the red terminal (copper pole) on the container. Attach the short black wire (with no plate attached to its end) to the black terminal (nickel pole) on the container and the other end to one of the terminals on top of the solution jar. The long black wire (with the large nickel plate) is attached to the other terminal on the solution jar. Both black wires (the short one and the long one) are thus attached to the terminals on the solution jar.

Now the plates at the ends of the wires are ready to be applied to your body. Place the small copper plate (on the red wire) to the designated spinal center, holding it in place with tape or a strap. Next, attach the large nickel plate (on the black wire) over the lacteal duct area: this is on the abdomen, three-finger widths to the right of the navel and one-finger width above the navel. (Lacteal ducts are lymphatic vessels in the small intestine.) Hold it in place with tape or a strap.

Lie down, relax, and meditate (or sleep) while attached to the device. You may also do constructive visualization or read inspirational literature during the session. Maintain a positive attitude throughout the procedure.

After each treatment, disconnect the wires and remove the plates, keeping them separated. Polish them, and then store them in separate containers (such as plastic sandwich bags). When possible, place the wires, plates, and the solution jar's lid out in the sun for a while in between uses, and store them separately afterward. Remove the lid of the solution jar and replace it with a plain lid. Clean the loop by washing it with water and drying it with a paper towel. The loop remains attached to the lid and may also be cleaned with a fine wire brush to remove the rest of the solution. Some solutions such as silver nitrate and gold chloride react chemically with the lead wires—destroying them—so you may want to use rubber gloves to protect your hands when cleaning them. Store the jar and lid until the next session. Again, the wires are cleaned and polished twenty minutes before the next use.

The plates, wires, and solution jar's lid with its wire loop may be placed in the sun for several hours in between uses, as mentioned earlier. All items of the appliance should be stored in a safe, dry place.

If you are using more than one kind of solution for the solution jar, you will need an extra jar to hold it, with an extra wire loop lid to screw on top of it. Each solution has its own jar and its own wire loop lid. Solution jars that carry a light-sensitive chemical such as gold chloride or silver nitrate may be covered with a black plastic tape to keep out the light, since light causes the solution to deteriorate too quickly. When using two solutions, alternate them; that is, use one solution one day and another the next day.

After every fourteen to fifteen uses, the solution jar should be dumped out, cleaned thoroughly, and changed, and a fresh solution added to the jar. Also clean the lead loop with fine emery paper. Every thirty days the whole appliance needs to be recharged. The contents of the container are dumped, the container is washed—as in the beginning—and the lead loop (on the solution jar's lid), the rods, and plates are cleansed with fine emery paper. A fresh mixture is added to the container, since the appliance probably will be reused for another thirty days. After its contents have been disposed of, the solution jar should also be refilled.

You might consider obtaining a large plastic chest with a matching lid to store the Wet-Cell and its accessories, leaving them in the chest until you dump out the chemicals after thirty days. The chest would help to keep all the materials in one place.

DIRECTIONS FROM THE READINGS

For a two-year-old girl with Down's syndrome (reading given on October 29, 1942):

There may be applications in which elements may be carried

vibratorially to the body that would supply energies to build brain centers. And we may see the demonstration here of those things that we have indicated through these channels, as to how there may be gradually built a brain—as to build near to normal reactions, with the ability of the body to develop normally in its physical, mental and spiritual natures—through the use of the low electrical vibrations, with the application of the mechanical therapy to centers from which there are radial activities to the central nerve system and to the sensory or sympathetic forces.

But this will require patience and persistence. However, it will give this entity, this body, an opportunity for its expression in this particular experience.

. . . Use the low Wet Cell Appliance for nerve energy building.

The Wet Cell Appliance would be used once each day for thirty minutes, preferably as the body sleeps.

The solution for charging the Wet Cell Appliance would be as follows; in the gallon and a half of distilled water:

Copper Sulphate	1½ pounds,
Sulphuric Acid C.P.	1 ounce,
Zinc	15 grains,
Willow Charcoal	½ pound.

The Appliance would carry a Gold Solution, the proportions being one grain Chloride of Gold to each ounce of Distilled Water; and use at least three ounces of the solution. Of course, change the Gold Solution after using fifteen days.

The attachments would be made in this manner:

The small copper plate would be attached to the 9th dorsal plexus, while the large nickel plate—through which the Gold Solution passes vibratorially—would be attached to the lacteal duct center, three fingers from the naval center to the right and one finger up . . .

Do these for thirty days—then we should give further instructions for the use of that to enable the body to build. These suggestions are merely the beginning, of course.   2836-1

TESTIMONIALS/RESULTS

In the July/August 1993 issue of *Venture Inward* magazine, Maybritt Hansen, a freelance writer, details her journey in the article "The Wet-Cell: Overcoming MS" (pp. 12–13, 45). At age thirty–seven, she was told she had multiple sclerosis (MS), a degenerative disease of the central nervous system. MS destroys the myelin sheath covering the nerves, resulting in poor transmission of messages from the brain to other parts of the body. She writes:

> "I have been using [the Wet-Cell Appliance] regularly for four months, and the progress in my condition is so remarkable that I again lead an active professional and social life. Few people know that I have any neurological irregularities at all. The Cayce appliance wasn't the only thing I used, but from the time I began using it, my progress accelerated noticeably . . .
>
> "I truly desired healing and believed that it would be mine. The Wet-Cell then supplied the needed vibrations to take my healing to this miraculous final stage . . .
>
> "If the Wet-Cell worked for me, it can work for anyone who truly wants to be well."

David Atkinson, whose book *Hope Springs Eternal: Surviving a Chronic Illness* (A.R.E. Press., 1998) describes his remarkable recovery from Lou Gehrig's disease (amyotrophic lateral sclerosis or ALS). He utilized a number of Cayce remedies, including the Wet–Cell Appliance. Amazingly in his fourteen–month recovery, he reversed his symptoms (first diagnosed in 1991)—unheard of in the medical community who disbelieved the diagnosis. Later, in 1997, a new test determined that his disease was specifically X-linked spinal bulbar muscular atrophy (SBMA), one of a subset of ailments that follows the ALS course of destroying nerves and one that is equally fatal. He traveled all over the U.S., volunteering his time and advice to inform others of the beneficial effects of the Cayce remedies. Atkinson passed away a few years ago.

ADDITIONAL INFORMATION

To help clarify "specifics" on the Wet–Cell Appliance, here is one excerpt from the readings describing the body's vibratory rate:

> . . . we find . . . the human body made up of electronic vibration, with each atom and element of the body, each organ and organism of same, having its electronic or unit of vibration necessary for the sustenance of, and equilibrium in, that particular organism. Each unit, then, being a cell or a unit of life in itself, with its capacity of reproducing itself by the first form or law as is known of reproduction, by division of same. When any force in any organ, any element of the body, becomes deficient in its ability to reproduce that equilibrium necessary for the sustenance of the physical existence and reproduction of same, the portion becomes deficient, deficient through electronic energy as is necessary. This may become by injury, by disease, received from external forces; received from internal forces by the lack of eliminations as are produced in the system, by the lack of other agencies to meet the requirements of same in body.   1800-4

Every particle of matter has its peculiar vibratory rate. If water, for example, is heated until it turns to steam, its vibratory rate or period of frequency has been altered. In the same manner, any strain or binding in the body causes incoordination, which also affects circulation and results in inflammation. The action of the Wet–Cell Appliance deals with a vibratory theory, and the device has been recommended in severe cases of incoordination of the nervous system and of glands. Because of the serious nature of many of these illnesses, applying the Wet–Cell and following consistently a particular regimen require a great deal of patience and persistence, as stated earlier.

Usually one feels nothing in particular when using the device, so it may be difficult to continue the application. " . . . No vibration will be experienced at the time of this being attached . . . " states reading 229-1, and it may take some time to see results. Accordingly, there is the need for patience and consistency when using the Wet–Cell Appliance.

Appendix

AGING/LONGEVITY

311-4 M. 28 April 11, 1931

... [if] the assimilations and the eliminations would be kept nearer *normal* in the human family, the days might be extended to whatever period as was so desired; for the system is builded by the assimilations of that it takes within, and is able to bring resuscitations so long as the eliminations do not hinder.

1548-3 F. 35 August 26, 1938

Remember, the body does gradually renew itself constantly. Do not look upon the conditions which have existed as not being able to be eradicated from the system ...

Hold to that *knowledge*—and don't think of it as just theory—that the body *can,* the body *does* renew itself!

244-2 M. 70 October 18, 1926

... Many of the organs and the conditions show the changes as come about by the natural, or *so called* natural conditions in changes as the body succumbs to the effects of age or usage in the system. Much of this may be overcome. (Man should live much longer than has been ordinarily given—and will!)

BIRTHMARK
573-1 F. Adult June 6, 1934

(Q) What caused the birthmark on my baby's [2595]'s arm? How may this be removed?
(A) By massaging it with an equal mixture of Olive Oil and Castor Oil it will be prevented from increasing. Marks on many bodies, as on this one, are for a purpose—and if a Life Reading would be given it would be seen that it has a purpose to perform in the affairs of those in its own surroundings and in many others. A mark!

CALLUSES
543-26 F. 29 December 15, 1937

(Q) What would most help the {calluses} on both feet?
(A) A real massage morning and evening with an equal combination of Olive Oil and Tincture of Myrrh. Heat the Oil to add the Myrrh. This massaged over such places morning and evening will be found to be most beneficial.

276-4 F. 15 February 16, 1933

(Q) What caused growth on foot, and what should be used if it repeats itself?
(A) This was from irritation; and that best for the reduction of same, as we find, would be a massage with baking soda which has been dampened with spirits of camphor. This will be good for anyone having callous places or any attendant growths on feet; for it will remove them entirely!

2555-1 F. 71 May 4, 1941

(Q) What should be done for bottoms of feet and toes?
(A) The removal of the pressures in the lumbar axis will remove a great deal of this pressure, and this tendency for calluses on portions of the feet.

But massage the feet each evening for five days, and then leave off, then begin again, and so on, with the equal combination of Olive Oil and Peanut Oil. Rub on all that will be absorbed. Then put a very light wrapping or stocking upon the feet. The next morning they may be bathed or cleansed in tepid water.

CLEANSING

243-7 F. 48 December 19, 1927

Just as a comparison—of a poor nature, but—a rotten apple left in a barrel may make all of these rotten; yet no matter how many sound ones are put about it, the rotten one will never be made sound.

... If a cell is left in the system that should be eliminated, or if it *is* of that condition of inactivity, then all the cells gathered about it cannot heal that cell. It *must* produce sufficient of the lymph, or leucocyte, that condition which will gather about it and move it out of the system, to let the new supply take its place!

440-2 M. 23 December 13, 1933

... For, *every* one—everybody—should take an internal bath occasionally, as well as an external one. They would all be better off if they would!

2524-5 M. 43 January 13, 1944

... Clear the body as you do the mind of those things that have been hindered. The things that hinder physically are the poor eliminations. Set up better eliminations in the body. This is why osteopathy and hydrotherapy come nearer to being the basis of all needed treatments for physical disabilities.

COLD COIN

1842-1 M. 32 March 14, 1939

Do not take this as being something of superstition, or as something that would be a good luck charm—but if the entity will wear about its person, or in its pocket, a metal that is carbon steel—preferably in the groin pocket—it will prevent, it will ionize the body—from its very vibrations—to resist cold, congestion, and those inclinations for disturbance with the mucous membranes of the throat and nasal passages.

COLDS
3546-1 F. 19 January 13, 1944
. . . Don't be too much in the open air at night. Don't get colds by wet feet or sitting in drafts, or being in crowds that make the body susceptible to the cold germ.

Do keep the feet warm . . .

CONSISTENT AND PERSISTENT
850-2 F. Adult April 24, 1935
Be consistent, but be persistent with those applications as suggested. Not as mere rote to be gotten through with, either in the breathing exercises or the massages that are to be given, but rather *seeing* that these are to accomplish that within the physical reactions for the body. For each activity has its own reaction, whether in the mental or the material world. By the proper attitude they may be accorded one with another, as cooperative influences; but if one is thinking one thing and doing another, then they must be combative one with another. Be not double-minded.

EPSOM SALTS PACKS/GRAPE POULTICES
261-19 M. 47 October 27, 1935
(Q) Do you prefer Epsom Salts Packs or the Grape Poultices?
(A) The Epsom Salts Packs are preferable at this time . . . There is not so much inflammation as a tendency for congestion, see? Hence the relaxation by the use of the Epsom Salts; while the Grape Poultices are rather to dissipate inflammation, see?

FEET
1771-3 F. 21 June 26, 1939
(Q) Would you recommend special foot exercise?
(A) It would be well if there would be this exercise night and morning;

night before retiring—but after the massage as indicated, see; and of morning just before putting on the hose—after the massage has been given:

Stand erect (without anything on the feet, of course). Then raise the arms, gently, slowly, over the head—directly over the head. Then gradually rise on the toes. Then, as the body relaxes or lowers itself, lower the hands also, the hands extending in front of the body. Then rock back upon the heels, with the hands extended sufficiently to strain or to exercise the bursa of the heel, or those portions of the heel *and* the arch, you see, to aid in strengthening. Doing this, together *with* the massage of the properties indicated through heel and arch, and especially over the frontal portions of the foot, we will bring better conditions for same.

1620-3 F. 45 December 14, 1938

(Q) What is the most effective treatment to follow to stop the progression of structural destruction in my feet?
(A) Rising upon the toes twice a day, morning and evening—upon arising and before retiring. Before putting on shoes and stockings of morning. Raise the arms, rocking back and forth on the heel and toe. Gradually, as the body raises up, raise the arms high also. Such an exercise is most beneficial.

3381-1 M. 32 December 1, 1943

(Q) What can be done to strengthen arches?
(A) The massage with the oil will be helpful. Also an exercise each day of a certain character would be well, of morning before the shoes are put on—before the oil massage is given, of course, but do this daily: Stand flat on the floor and spring on the toes, rising gently and springing.

HAIR AND SCALP

257-227 M. 47 November 15, 1940

(Q) What will aid condition of hair and scalp?
(A) If you would seek that as would be of the *most* aid—drink the juice

from potato peelings about once or twice a week; and then massage the scalp with a weakened solution of Atomidine (a few drops to a tablespoonful of water). (Stew the potato peelings in a little water and drink.)

HALITOSIS

5198-1 F. 38 May 31, 1944

(Q) How can I get rid of bad breath?

(A) By making for better conditions in eliminations. Take Glyco-Thymoline as an intestinal antiseptic. Two, three times a day. Put six drops of Glyco-Thymoline in the water. This is a throwing off into the lung, into the body-forces, poisons from this changing in cellular activity, or through the body, of lymph forces that become fecal.

HEALING

1173-6 M. 28 November 14, 1936

. . . For after all, all *healing* is from the divine within, and not from medications. Medications only *attune* or accord a body for the proper reactions from the elemental forces of divinity within each corpuscle, each cell, each muscle, each activity of every atom of the body itself.

1173-8 M. 28 November 30, 1936

. . . For no element outside of body produces healing, but that the attunement to the coordinating and cooperative forces of life-force as it meets the various influences that have been brought about by some error or some misapplication, the awareness of the God-Force, the Life-Force working in and through the system.

These are the manners in which healing, in which enlightenment, in which knowledge comes to the applicable experience of the individual entity.

2930-1 M. Adult March 7, 1943

(Q) What is the best and quickest way to build up my health?

(A) As indicated, the mental attitudes—combined with the proper eliminations being kept. This will include exercises, of course, as well as the establishing of coordination in all of the eliminating channels of the body.

HEMORRHOIDS

2823-2 F. 33 June 5, 1943

(Q) What treatment should be followed for hemorrhoids?

(A) The best is to treat the general condition as indicated. But the best for the specific condition of hemorrhoids is the exercise, and if this is taken regularly these will disappear—of themselves! Twice each day, of morning and evening—and this doesn't mean with many clothes on! Rise on the toes, at the same time raising the arms; then bend forward, letting the hands go toward the floor. Do this three times of morning and three times of evening. But don't do it two or three times and then quit! Or don't do it three to four times a week and then quit, but do it regularly! Be regular with it, each day!

HYDROTHERAPY

257-254 M. 50 December 18, 1943

(Q) How often should the hydrotherapy be given?

(A) Dependent upon the general conditions. Whenever there is a sluggishness, the feeling of heaviness, oversleepiness, the tendency for an achy, draggy feeling, then have the treatments. This does not mean that merely because there is the daily activity of the alimentary canal there is no need for flushing the system. But whenever there is the feeling of sluggishness, have the treatments. It'll pick the body up. For there is a need for such treatments when the condition of the body becomes drugged because of absorption of poisons through alimentary canal or colon, sluggishness of liver or kidneys, and there is the lack of coordination with the cerebrospinal and sympathetic blood supply and nerves. For the hydrotherapy and massage are preventive as well as curative measures. For the cleansing of the system allows the body-forces themselves to function normally, and thus eliminate poisons, congestions and conditions that would become acute through the body.

635-9 F. 56 December 11, 1937

As we find for this body, the Hydrotherapy Bath would be well; which would be to lie in great quantities or a tub of water for a long period—this being kept a little above the temperature of the body; then followed by a thorough massage by a masseuse. This would be better than adjustments *or* deep treatments, though it will be found that with the massage along the spine, with the body prone upon the face, these would—with the knuckle on either side of the spinal column—tend to make many a segment come nearer to normalcy, by being so treated *after* having been thoroughly relaxed for twenty to thirty minutes *in* the warm or hot water, see?

IMMUNIZATION

1958-4 F. 4 September 8, 1943

(Q) What will immune the body against Infantile Paralysis?

(A) Nothing will immune the body if it comes in contact with the conditions, but the extra quantity of iodine (as in the Atomidine, which is atomic iodine) should keep the glands purified so that the body may be in a better condition to be immune . . .

(Q) Would it be well to vaccinate the body for Smallpox now or wait until next Spring?

(A) Don't do it while the blood is in its present condition. You might do it after the body has been taking the Atomidine and the Calcios for at least a month or six weeks, and then it would be in a good fix for vaccination.

INTENTION

2415-2 F. Adult December 5, 1940

. . . Do not make the application in a way, however, that it is just something to be gotten through with, or rid of, but do it with the intent and the expectation that it is to be a helpful experience for the body; and it will! . . .

LAXATIVES

286-8 F. Adult September 27, 1940

Be mindful that there is not allowed to be a day without proper eliminations. Do not overtake cathartics or laxatives. Use rather small doses
of Olive Oil often—that is, about a quarter to half a teaspoonful taken
several times during a day.

MOLES

573-1 F. Adult June 6, 1934

(Q) What treatment would remove the mole on my chest, or is this
advisable?

(A) Haven't we just given it? The massage with the Castor Oil twice
each day; not rubbing hard, but *gentle* massage around and over the
place. And it will be removed. [Miss Wynne reported on March 9, 1935,
that mole had entirely disappeared.]

4033-2 F. 62 August 25, 1944

(Q) What should be done for the small mole or soft growth on left side
of back, just below the shoulder blade, that gets irritated at times and
is painful?

(A) Use a small quantity of Castor Oil with a little soda mixed in same.
This will make it sore for a day or two, then it will disappear.

(Q) Just rub it on?

(A) Just rub it on, two or three days apart, for two or three times.

NAILS

3025-1 F. 45 May 27, 1943

(Q) What should be done for breaking of nails?

(A) We would massage the fingers around the cuticle with the
Atomidine. This will tend to color for a while, but with the treatments
that have been indicated, and the rubs, and the diets—with this used
once or twice a week so as to allow that already begun to grow, we
should have better condition of the nails.

POISON IVY

261-33 M. 51 August 29, 1938

As we find, the specific or acute conditions arising as a rash are the effects of contact with poison ivy.

We would for this particular disturbance in the present:

Bathe off the affected parts with a weak solution of Atomidine; the proportions being about a teaspoonful to half a glass of water. Sponge off same with a tuft of cotton.

PROGNOSIS

5671-7 F. 34 January 13, 1930

(Q) How many days from today will body be cured?

(A) That depends upon the response of the body. That is the same as that of swatting the fly! . . .

The body is doing well. Only be a little patient. Just know that, will the body keep itself in as close attunement to those applications being made as is possible, it will grow—with the reliefs as are brought for physical reactions in the system. Be a little patient, be very persistent, and also consistent . . .

PYORRHEA

5121-1 F. 52 May 17, 1944

(Q) What can I do about pyorrhea condition in my teeth?

(A) Use Ipsab regularly each day and rinse mouth out when it is finished with Glyco-Thymoline. Massage gums inside and out by wetting a small tuft of cotton with the Ipsab or use the finger alone, and massage with the Ipsab. It will remove and correct the conditions . . .

3696-1 F. 31 March 16, 1944

The receding gums and those tendencies towards pyorrhea would be allayed by the consistent use of Ipsab as a massage for the teeth and gums. Also these should be treated, some locally, with the dentist's paraphernalia—the small wads of cotton saturated with the Ipsab and applied in the areas where the conditions are indicated at the base or edge of the gums.

SCAR TISSUE

4003-1 M. 45 March 24, 1944

... {*After the Epsom salts packs*} massage the limb and foot with cocoa butter. Do not break up the deposits of the scar tissue, or calcium deposits, more than can be regularly or naturally done by increasing the eliminations; that is, do not break up more of the scar tissue than can be eliminated from the body. These should be eliminated not only through the respiratory and perspiratory system but through the alimentary canal . . . .

SNEEZING

816-8 M. 53 January 20, 1937

(Q) Occasionally the membranes in the nose become sensitive, the body starts sneezing, and a cold develops. At such times can anything be done to soothe the membranes and stop the sneezing?

(A) A weak solution of Atomidine; teaspoonful of Atomidine to an ounce of distilled water, used as a spray, will retard—and build for normalcy in irritations as produced by cold germ. This may arise as much from anger or anxiety mentally as from cold or congestion, however.

TAPEWORMS

567-7 M. 26 February 27, 1935

If there is the desire on the part of the body to test self for tape worms, live for three days on raw apples *only!* Then take about half a teacup of olive oil, or half a glass of olive oil. And this would remove fecal matter that hasn't been removed for some time! But it will certainly indicate there is no tape worm.

TEETH

457-11 F. 34 September 3, 1942

(Q) What causes the gray film on teeth?

(A) The chemical balance in the system and the throw-off or discharge from breath in the lungs. This is a source from which drosses are relieved from the system, and thus passing through the teeth produce same on the teeth. Keeping such cleansed with an equal combination of soda and salt at least three to four times a week will cleanse these of this disturbance. The use of Ipsab as a wash for mouth and gums will further aid in keeping these conditions cleansed; and any good dentifrice once or twice a day.

3484-1 M. 40 December 27, 1943

(Q) What is best procedure for care of teeth?
(A) Have local attention and then take care of the teeth. Use an equal combination of salt and soda for massaging the gums and teeth—don't use a brush, use your finger!

3436-1 M. 45 November 30, 1943

(Q) What can I do to keep my teeth for life?
(A) You won't! For already these have begun to need local attention. If there is kept the proper balance in the vitamins, it will help—but these precautions should begin—well, during the period of gestation is when they should begin, but for a body should begin at least in the first or second year.

325-55 F. 62 January 24, 1925

(Q) Does gold in mouth help to cause bitterness?
(A) It does! No teeth should ever be filled with heavy metals, as gold. Much preferable would be the compositions that make themselves one with the properties themselves; much preferable.

TOXEMIA

464-31 F. 65 February 21, 1941

(Q) Please advise as to nerves, high blood pressure and intestinal trouble.
(A) All of these have been covered in that indicated. For, all of these are results from this toxic condition which arises from pressures in the spinal system which have needed correction, and which have never been fully corrected. Then, when other disturbances arise—such as cold, congestion, overanxiety, anger, indigestion—all of these then

become problems to be taken care of in the system; so that they do leave the toxic poisons.

(Q) What is the toxic poisoning and what produces it?

(A) As just given. The word toxic itself means poison, but poison is not always toxic!

When there is the lack of eliminations of used energies, or of refuse or carbon as it might be called, or the ash of nerve and muscular forces still left in the system, it becomes toxic poison—or toxemia.

Toxic poison, then, is that condition in alimentary canal, in liver, kidneys, throughout the circulation repressing the activities—owing to the quantity of ash left from body refuse not eliminated.

WARNINGS

1861-11 M. 35 January 30, 1942

As to the violet ray application—there has been indicated a specific time. This has been overstepped at times, with the idea that if a little would do good more would do more good; while at times more does harm rather than good! It is as an overtaxation even to a strong muscular force may weaken, may even deter the best activity. Do not overstrain, but keep the violet ray—and not more than the minute and a half. Two to three minutes is worse than none being given!

WARTS

308-13 F. 70 June 26, 1944

(Q) What is the best way to remove warts?

(A) This one on the right knee is gradually leaving. Put equal portions of Castor Oil and Soda on the finger tip, massage this, it'll make it sore but it'll take it away also.

1179-4 F. 9 November 24, 1937

(Q) How can [1179] get rid of her warts?

(A) Apply a paste of baking soda with Castor Oil. Mix together and apply of evenings. Just the proportions so it makes almost a *gum;* not as dough but more as gum, see? A pinch between the fingers with three to four drops in the palm of the hand, and this worked together and then placed on—bound on. It may make for irritation after the second or third application, but leave it off for one evening and then apply the next—and it will be disappearing!

WHOOPING COUGH/PNEUMONIA

5671-16 F. 34 May 10, 1930

(Q) Can the body give her baby anything for the whooping cough?

(A) That as has been outlined for whooping cough. Can give it anything, but this would be helpful—as has been outlined for same through these same suggestions. Use occasionally a few drops of the Syrup of Squill—three to five drops may be given two or three times a day. When the cough is severe, give five to ten drops of *kerosene*—in sugar or plain. *Massage* the body thoroughly—especially through the upper dorsal region—with equal parts of olive oil and tincture of myrrh. Heat the oil and add the myrrh. *This* will relieve the condition. When the nausea comes, if there is given the juice of onions—not with that that is boiled in water, but heated and the juice pressed out—this is the best thing for pneumonia that may be given!

Symptom: Remedy

A

Abdominal pain
Grape poultice

Abrasions
Castor oil, massage, mullein stupe, Violet Ray (skin), Wet–Cell Appliance

Aches
Epsom salts bath

Acidity
Apple diet, Atomidine, castor oil pack, Glyco–Thymoline, olive oil, warm/hot water beverage

Adenoiditis
Onion juice

Adhesions
Apple cider vinegar, apple diet, castor oil pack, Epsom salts pack, grape poultice, onion poultice (lung), sand pack, steam/fume bath, Wet–Cell Appliance

Alcoholism
Radio–Active Appliance, Wet–Cell Appliance

Alzheimer's disease
  Wet–Cell Appliance
Amyotrophic lateral sclerosis (ALS)
  Wet–Cell Appliance
Anemia
  Apple diet, beef juice, liver juice (pernicious), Radio–Active Appliance, sand pack
Anxiety
  Violet Ray
Aphonia
  Castor oil pack
Apoplexy
  Peanut oil massage
Appendicitis
  Castor oil pack, grape poultice, Radio–Active Appliance
Appetite control
  Grape juice
Appetite (poor)
  Red wine with black bread
Arthritis
  Apple cider vinegar, apple diet, Atomidine, castor oil pack, hot packs (not for rheumatoid), Epsom salts bath, Epsom salts pack, massage, peanut oil massage, Radio–Active Appliance, sand pack, sitz bath, steam/fume bath, Violet Ray, Wet–Cell Appliance
Assimilation
  See Poor assimilations
Asthenia
  Olive oil
Asthma
  Atomidine, breathing exercises, charred oak keg, onion poultice, Wet–Cell Appliance
Attempting conception
  Myrrh

B

Backache
Electric vibrator, turpentine

Bad breath
See Halitosis

Baldness
Alternating hot and cold packs, Atomidine, electric vibrator, Violet Ray

Bed soreness
Myrrh

Better sleep
Violet Ray

Bites
Atomidine, Glyco-Thymoline

Bladder ailments
Glyco-Thymoline, mullein stupe, turpentine (for infection)

Bladder stricture
Turpentine

Blemishes (on skin)
Peanut oil massage

Blepharitis
Potato poultice

Blindness
Potato poultice, Wet-Cell Appliance

Blood building
Liver juice

Body strengthener
Beef juice, grape juice, liver juice

Boils
Atomidine, mullein stupe

Brain disorders
Wet-Cell Appliance

Brain lesion
Head and neck exercise

Brain tumor
Wet-Cell Appliance
Breast tumor
Wet-Cell Appliance
Broken bones
Apple cider vinegar
Bronchiectasis
Charred oak keg
Bronchitis
Apple diet, charred oak keg, head and neck exercise, onion juice, onion poultice
Bruised tendons
Apple cider vinegar
Bruises
Epsom salts bath, mullein stupe
Build up resistance
Beef juice
Bumps (on skin)
Peanut oil massage
Bunions
Massage
Burns
Glyco-Thymoline, peanut oil massage, Wet-Cell Appliance
Bursitis
Hot pack

C

Calcium deficiency
Beef juice
Calluses
Myrrh, turpentine (on feet)
Cancer
Beef juice, castor oil pack, mullein stupe, Violet Ray, Wet-Cell Appliance

Cartilage misalignment
Apple cider vinegar
Cataracts
Breathing exercises, head and neck exercise, potato poultice, steam/fume bath, Violet Ray
Catarrh
Epsom salts bath, Glyco-Thymoline, head and neck exercise, onion juice, Radio-Active Appliance
Cerebral hemorrhage
Apple diet, Wet-Cell Appliance
Cerebral palsy
Castor oil pack, Radio-Active Appliance, sand pack, Wet-Cell Appliance
Chapped skin
Glyco-Thymoline
Chest pain
Violet Ray
Childbirth (aftereffects)
Apple diet, Epsom salts pack
Cholecystalgia
Castor oil pack
Cholecystitis
Alternating hot and cold packs, castor oil pack, peanut oil massage
Chronic obstructive pulmonary disease
Charred oak keg
Circulation problems
See Poor circulation
Cirrhosis of the liver
Castor oil pack, Wet-Cell Appliance
Cold feet
Radio-Active Appliance, Violet Ray
Cold prevention
Atomidine, Epsom salts bath
Colds
Charred oak keg, coffee foot bath, Glyco-Thymoline, hot pack, olive

oil, onion juice, onion poultice, Radio–Active Appliance, steam/fume bath, turpentine

Colitis

Apple cider vinegar, castor oil pack, Epsom salts pack, grape poultice, olive oil, sand pack, Wet–Cell Appliance

Color blindness

Wet–Cell Appliance

Congestion

Coffee foot bath, electric vibrator (throat and head), Glyco–Thymoline, onion juice, onion poultice, Radio–Active Appliance, steam/fume bath, turpentine

Conjunctivitis

Potato poultice

Constipation

Apple diet, castor oil pack, massage, olive oil, sitz bath, warm/hot water beverage

Coronary occlusion

Peanut oil massage

Coughs

Breathing exercises, charred oak keg

Cramping (hands and feet)

Myrrh

Cuts

Atomidine

Cystitis

Sitz bath, turpentine

Cysts

Atomidine, castor oil pack, myrrh

D

Deafness

Head and neck exercise (tendency toward), Radio–Active Appliance, Wet–Cell Appliance

Debilitation (general)

Apple diet, beef juice, liver juice, myrrh, onion juice, peanut oil massage, Radio–Active Appliance, red wine with black bread, sand pack, showers, Wet–Cell Appliance

Dental problems
Atomidine

Denture cleaning
Glyco-Thymoline

Depression
Showers, Wet–Cell Appliance

Dermatitis
Mullein stupe, peanut oil massage, Wet–Cell Appliance

Detoxing
Head and neck exercise, steam/fume bath

Diabetes
Wet–Cell Appliance

Diarrhea
Castor oil pack

Digestion problems
Epsom salts pack, Glyco-Thymoline, olive oil, Radio–Active Appliance, turpentine, Violet Ray, warm/hot water beverage

Dilation of the abdomen
Mullein stupe

Dizziness
Atomidine, electric vibrator, mullein tea

Down's syndrome
Wet–Cell Appliance

Dry skin
Massage, olive oil, peanut oil massage, Violet Ray

Dry throat
Breathing exercises

Dysmenorrhea
Myrrh, sitz bath, turpentine, Violet Ray

E

Earache
Violet Ray

Ear problems
Glyco-Thymoline, head and neck exercise
Eczema
Sand pack
Edema (*see also* Swelling)
Mullein stupe
Elephantiasis
Breathing exercises
Eliminations
See Poor eliminations
Emphysema
Charred oak keg
Enlarged joints
Radio-Active Appliance
Enteritis
Epsom salts pack
Epilepsy
Apple diet, beef juice, castor oil pack, peanut oil massage, Radio-Active Appliance, sand pack, Wet-Cell Appliance
Excessive hair
Atomidine
Excessive mucus
Turpentine
Exhaustion
Steam/fume bath, Violet Ray
Eye discoloration
Showers
Eye lesions
Potato poultice
Eyelid irritations
Potato poultice (granulated lids)
Eye problems
Glyco-Thymoline, head and neck exercise, potato poultice (infection, inflammation), Violet Ray, Wet-Cell Appliance

Eyes (burning, tired)
Potato poultice
Eyesight (poor)
Potato poultice
Eyestrain
Violet Ray, warm/hot water beverage

F

Facial tic
Alternating hot and cold packs
Fading hair color
Violet Ray
Fatigue
Beef juice, breathing exercises, castor oil pack, coffee foot bath, Epsom salts bath, myrrh, peanut oil massage, showers, sitz bath
Feet
Epsom salts pack, Radio–Active Appliance (cold)
Feminine hygiene
Atomidine
Fever
Cold pack, massage, olive oil, onion poultice
Fibrosis
Charred oak keg
Fingernails
Apple cider vinegar, Atomidine
Fistulas
Epsom salts pack (womb, vagina), sitz bath
Flatulence
Castor oil pack, grape juice, grape poultice
Flu
See Influenza
Flu-like symptoms
Beef juice
Food poisoning
Grape poultice

Fractures
Apple cider vinegar, onion poultice (ribs)
Frequent urination
Radio–Active Appliance
Fresh injury
Cold pack
Fullness in throat and head
Steam/fume bath

G

Gain weight
Beef juice
Gallstones
Castor oil pack
Gastritis
Castor oil pack, Epsom salts pack, grape poultice
Generative conditions
Radio–Active Appliance
Glandular disorders (incoordination)
Atomidine, beef juice, Epsom salts pack, grape poultice, head and neck exercise, peanut oil massage, Wet–Cell Appliance
Glaucoma
Wet–Cell Appliance
Goiter
Atomidine, breathing exercises, Glyco–Thymoline, Radio–Active Appliance, Violet Ray (tendency), Wet–Cell Appliance
Gout
Hot pack
Grating knee and hip bone
Sitz bath
Gynecological problems
Myrrh

H

Hair disorders
Violet Ray
Hair growth
Violet Ray
Halitosis
Castor oil pack, Glyco-Thymoline
Hangnails
Atomidine
Hard nails
Atomidine
Hay fever
Charred oak keg
Headaches
Apple diet, castor oil pack, electric vibrator, Epsom salts bath, head and neck exercise, massage, showers, Violet Ray, Wet-Cell Appliance (migraines)
Head noises
Head and neck exercise, sand pack
Hearing difficulties
Head and neck exercise, olive oil
Hearing loss
Massage
Heart condition
Peanut oil massage
Heaviness
Breathing exercises (across small of back), coffee foot bath (in throat, head, and feet)
Hemorrhaging
Electric vibrator
Hemorrhoids
Epsom salts pack, sitz bath
Hepatitis
Castor oil pack

Hernias
  Castor oil pack, myrrh, showers
Hives
  Mullein tea
Hoarseness
  Electric vibrator
Hodgkin's disease
  Castor oil pack
Hookworm
  Castor oil pack
Hypertension
  Apple diet, Atomidine, castor oil pack, Radio-Active Appliance, Wet-Cell Appliance
Hyperthyroidism
  Breathing exercises

I

Ichthyosis
  Castor oil
Immune system (low)
  Red wine with black bread
Impaired locomotion
  Alternating hot and cold packs, Epsom salts bath, Epsom salts pack, olive oil, peanut oil massage
Impaired speech
  Breathing exercises
Incoordination (between sympathetic and cerebrospinal nervous systems)
  Wet-Cell Appliance
Infantile paralysis
  Atomidine, Wet-Cell Appliance
Infection
  Atomidine, Epsom salts pack
Infertility
  Alternating hot and cold packs

Inflammation
Atomidine, castor oil pack, cold pack, grape poultice, mullein stupe
Influenza
Epsom salts bath, Epsom salts pack, hot pack, onion poultice, sitz bath
Ingrown toenails
Atomidine
Injuries
Apple cider vinegar, cold pack (fresh), Epsom salts bath, Epsom salts pack, grape poultice, mullein stupe, onion poultice (from a fall), steam/fume bath
Insomnia
Atomidine, electric vibrator, massage, Radio-Active Appliance, steam/fume bath, Violet Ray, Wet-Cell Appliance
Intestinal impaction
Castor oil pack
Intestinal inflammation
Mullein tea
Intestinal problems
Cold pack, Epsom salts pack, Glyco-Thymoline, grape juice, Radio-Active Appliance
Intestinal worms
Apple diet
Iritis
Wet-Cell Appliance
Itching
Myrrh (abdomen), olive oil (scalp), sitz bath (thighs, legs, vulva), Violet Ray (scalp)

J

Joint pain
Apple cider vinegar, Epsom salts bath, hot pack, massage, showers
Joints
Radio-Active Appliance

K

Kidneys
Epsom salts pack, turpentine (infection)
Kidney stones
Mullein stupe, mullein tea, turpentine

L

Lacerations
Steam/fume bath
Leg pain
Electric vibrator, massage
Leg twitching
Massage
Lesions
Alternating hot and cold packs (psoriasis-like), apple cider vinegar, castor oil pack, Epsom salts bath, Epsom salts pack, grape poultice, potato poultice (eye), sand pack, steam/fume bath
Leukemia
Atomidine, Radio-Active Appliance
Liver
Castor oil pack, Epsom salts pack
Liver and stomach pain
Atomidine
Lou Gehrig's disease (ALS)
Wet-Cell Appliance
Low immune system
Red wine with black bread
Low stamina/vitality
Beef juice, peanut oil massage
Lumbago
Apple cider vinegar, Epsom salts bath, Epsom salts pack, sand pack
Lumbar strain
Myrrh
Lung adhesions
Onion poultice

Lung congestion
Charred oak keg, electric vibrator
Lymphatic disturbances
Grape poultice
Lymphitis
Castor oil pack
Lymph tumor
Wet–Cell Appliance

M

Mastoiditis
Head and neck exercise
Measles
Onion poultice
Melancholia
Showers
Memory (poor)
Radio–Active Appliance
Menopause
Apple diet, massage, peanut oil massage, Radio–Active Appliance, sitz bath
Menstrual cramps
Radio-Active Appliance, showers
Menstrual irregularity
Radio-Active Appliance
Menstrual period
Epsom salts pack (prior to)
Menstruation problems
Atomidine
Mental disorders
Wet–Cell Appliance
Migraine headaches
Wet–Cell Appliance
Moles
Castor oil

Mouth sores
Atomidine

Mucosity
Glyco–Thymoline, turpentine

Multiple sclerosis
Beef juice, castor oil pack, peanut oil massage, Wet–Cell Appliance

Muscle aches
Epsom salts bath, hot pack, massage, myrrh, steam/fume bath

Muscle atrophy
Mullein stupe, Wet–Cell Appliance

Muscle contractions
Massage

Muscles
Epsom salts pack, massage, peanut oil massage (sore, tight), steam/fume bath (sore)

Muscle spasms
Cold pack, electric vibrator, massage, Wet–Cell Appliance

Muscle strain
Massage

Muscular dystrophy
Wet–Cell Appliance

Myopia
Head and neck exercise, potato poultice

N

Nasal drip
Charred oak keg

Nausea
Castor oil pack, Radio–Active Appliance, warm/hot water beverage

Neck and forehead (to cool during warm treatments)
Cold pack

Neck carbuncles
Atomidine

Need for better rest
Coffee foot bath

Need for stimulant
Red wine with black bread
Nephritis
Sitz bath
Nerve endings (impaired, atrophied)
Wet-Cell Appliance
Nerve exhaustion
Electric vibrator
Nervousness
Head and neck exercise, massage, Radio-Active Appliance
Nervous system incoordination
Alternating hot and cold packs, apple diet, castor oil pack, Epsom salts bath, head and neck exercise, peanut oil massage, Radio-Active Appliance, sand pack, showers, Violet Ray
Neuralgia
Epsom salts pack, hot pack
Neurasthenia
Apple diet, Radio-Active Appliance, sand pack, Wet-Cell Appliance
Neuritis
Apple cider vinegar, apple diet, Atomidine, castor oil pack, Epsom salts bath, Epsom salts pack, peanut oil massage, Radio-Active Appliance, steam/fume bath, Wet-Cell Appliance
Neurosis
Myrrh, sand pack
Night sweats
Massage
Nodules
Atomidine
Noises in head
Sand pack
Numbness
Epsom salts pack (fingers and toes), peanut oil massage (in legs)

O

Obesity
Grape juice, Radio-Active Appliance, Wet-Cell Appliance
Oral hygiene
Glyco-Thymoline
Osteochondritis
Head and neck exercise
Overtaxation
Electric vibrator

P

Painful areas
Cold pack, Epsom salts pack, mullein stupe, steam/fume bath, Violet
Ray (chest)
Painful menstruation
See Dysmenorrhea
Painful urination
Radio-Active Appliance
Palsy
Peanut oil massage
Paralysis
Epsom salts bath, Epsom salts pack, Wet-Cell Appliance
Parkinson's disease
Castor oil pack, liver juice, Wet-Cell Appliance
Peeling skin on feet
Coffee foot bath, massage
Pelvic cellulitis
Apple cider vinegar, castor oil pack, myrrh
Pelvic disorders
Apple diet, breathing exercises, Epsom salts pack, head and neck ex-
ercise, sitz bath, steam/fume bath
Peritonitis
Grape juice, grape poultice
Personal hygiene
Glyco-Thymoline

Phlebitis
Mullein stupe
Pinworms
Apple diet
Pleurisy
Charred oak keg, onion poultice, steam/fume bath
Pneumonia
Charred oak keg, onion juice, onion poultice
Poison ivy
Atomidine, Glyco–Thymoline
Polio
Peanut oil massage
Poor appetite
Red wine with black bread
Poor assimilations (incoordination)
Apple diet, beef juice, breathing exercises, grape poultice, myrrh, red wine with black bread, warm/hot water beverage
Poor circulation
Breathing exercises, castor oil pack, coffee foot bath, Epsom salts bath, head and neck exercise, mullein stupe, mullein tea, onion juice, peanut oil massage, Radio–Active Appliance, sand pack, showers, sitz bath, Violet Ray, Wet–Cell Appliance
Poor eliminations (incoordination)
Apple diet, beef juice, castor oil pack, coffee foot bath, Epsom salts pack, grape juice, grape poultice, head and neck exercise, myrrh, olive oil, peanut oil massage, red wine with black bread, sand pack, sitz bath, steam/fume bath, turpentine, Violet Ray, warm/hot water beverage, Wet–Cell Appliance
Poor eyesight
Electric vibrator, massage, potato poultice, turpentine
Poor memory
Radio–Active Appliance
Post–nasal drip
Glyco–Thymoline

Post–surgery
  Massage
Pregnancy
  Massage, sitz bath
Prenatal conditions
  Radio–Active Appliance
Prolapsis
  Castor oil pack, Epsom salts bath
Prostatitis
  Sitz bath, Wet–Cell Appliance
Protuberance
  Radio–Active Appliance
Pruritus vulvae
  Myrrh, sitz bath
Psoriasis–like lesions
  Alternating hot and cold packs
Ptomaine poisoning
  Grape poultice

R

Rashes
  Atomidine, peanut oil massage, showers
Recklinghausen's disease
  Grape poultice, mullein stupe, Wet–Cell Appliance
Recuperation
  Liver juice
Relaxation
  Olive oil (prior to adjustments), steam/fume bath (need for)
Renal calculus
  Turpentine
Reproductive organ disorders
  Violet Ray
Respiratory problems
  Turpentine

Restlessness
Electric vibrator, Violet Ray

Retardation
Wet-Cell Appliance

Retinitis pigmentosa
Potato poultice, sand pack

Rheumatism
Apple cider vinegar, Epsom salts bath, Epsom salts pack, grape poultice, peanut oil massage, Radio-Active Appliance, Violet Ray

Rheumatoid arthritis
Wet-Cell Appliance

Riggs's disease
Violet Ray

Ringing in head and ears
Peanut oil massage

Ringworm
Castor oil pack, Violet Ray, Wet-Cell Appliance

S

Sarcoidosis
Charred oak keg

Sarcoma
Epsom salts pack

Scaly, tough skin
Atomidine, Violet Ray (scalp)

Scars on lungs
Breathing exercises

Sciatica
Epsom salts bath, Epsom salts pack, Wet-Cell Appliance

Scleroderma
Castor oil pack, Epsom salts bath, Wet-Cell Appliance

Senility
Radio-Active Appliance, Wet-Cell Appliance

Shortness of breath
Breathing exercises, charred oak keg, electric vibrator

Sinus irritation

Atomidine, Violet Ray

Sinusitis

Breathing exercises, Epsom salts pack, Glyco-Thymoline, head and neck exercise

Skin cancer

Grape poultice

Skin conditions

Steam/fume bath, Violet Ray (abrasions), Wet-Cell Appliance (dermatitis)

Skin eruptions

Atomidine

Sluggish eliminations

Alternating hot and cold packs

Sluggish liver

Castor oil pack, sand pack

Sluggish thyroid

Atomidine

Smoker's lung

Charred oak keg

Soften hard areas

Epsom salts pack

Soreness

Atomidine, peanut oil massage (muscles)

Sore throat

Atomidine

Speaking difficulties

Head and neck exercise

Speech, impaired

Breathing exercises

Spinal misalignment (subluxation)

Apple cider vinegar, apple diet, electric vibrator, Epsom salts pack, Glyco-Thymoline (prior to adjustments), head and neck exercise, hot pack, myrrh, Radio-Active Appliance, sand pack

Split fingernails
   Atomidine
Sprains
   Apple cider vinegar, Epsom salts bath, hot pack
Stenosis of the duodenum
   Castor oil pack
Sterility
   Castor oil pack, Wet–Cell Appliance
Stiff joints
   Massage, peanut oil massage, sitz bath
Stiff muscles/limbs
   Atomidine, Epsom salts bath, massage, sitz bath
Stiff neck
   Massage
Stings
   Glyco–Thymoline
Stomach ulcer
   Peanut oil massage
Strains
   Apple cider vinegar, hot pack, myrrh
Strangulation of kidneys
   Castor oil pack
Streptococcus
   Breathing exercises
Stress
   Head and neck exercise, massage, peanut oil massage, Radio–Active
   Appliance, showers
Stricture of the duodenum
   Castor oil pack
Stroke
   Apple diet, peanut oil massage
Sunburn
   Apple cider vinegar, Glyco–Thymoline
Surgery (aftereffects)
   Beef juice

Swallowing difficulties

Violet Ray

Swelling

Castor oil pack, massage, mullein stupe, peanut oil massage (feet)

Swollen joints/glands

Atomidine

T

Tender skin (on back)

Myrrh

Tension

Myrrh

Throat irritations

Glyco–Thymoline, onion juice

Tic douloureux

Epsom salts pack

Tinnitus

Head and neck exercise

Tonsillitis

Head and neck exercise, onion juice, onion poultice

Tooth decay

Atomidine

Torn ligaments

Apple cider vinegar

Torticollis

Radio–Active Appliance, Wet–Cell Appliance

Toxemia

Alternating hot and cold packs, apple diet, castor oil pack, electric vibrator, Epsom salts bath, Epsom salts pack, grape juice, olive oil, onion poultice, peanut oil massage, sand pack, showers, sitz bath, steam/fume bath, Wet–Cell Appliance

Tuberculosis/TB of bone

Apple cider vinegar, beef juice, breathing exercises, charred oak keg, grape poultice, onion juice, onion poultice, sand pack, sitz bath

Tumors

Atomidine, beef juice, castor oil pack, Epsom salts pack, grape poultice, myrrh, sand pack, Wet–Cell Appliance

Typhoid fever

Grape poultice

U

Ulcers

Grape poultice, peanut oil massage (stomach), Wet–Cell Appliance

Uremia

Castor oil pack, Epsom salts pack

Urination (frequent, painful)

Radio–Active Appliance

Uterine fibroid tumor

Violet Ray, Wet–Cell Appliance

Uterus

Epsom salts pack

V

Vaginal fistulas

Castor oil pack

Vaginal irritations

Sitz bath

Vaginal pains

Turpentine

Vaginitis

Myrrh, Radio–Active Appliance

Varicose veins

Head and neck exercise, massage, mullein stupe, mullein tea, peanut oil massage

Venereal disease

Atomidine, Epsom salts bath (aftereffects), sitz bath, Wet–Cell Appliance

Vertigo

Atomidine, head and neck exercise, Wet–Cell Appliance

Vision problems
  Potato poultice, Radio–Active Appliance
Vitiligo
  Wet–Cell Appliance
Vulvitis
  Apple cider vinegar

W

Warts
  Castor oil
Weak arches (feet)
  Coffee foot bath, massage
Weakness
  Beef juice, peanut oil massage (knees, legs), red wine with black bread
Weak uterine walls
  Myrrh
Weight gain
  Beef juice
Wens
  Castor oil
Whooping cough
  Onion juice
Wilms' tumor
  Epsom salts pack

BIBLIOGRAPHY

Adelglass, Dr. Howard. "Heat a Backache? Cool a Sprain?" *Today's Focus* (for the Associated Press): n.d.

Barron, Patrick, NMD. *Hydrotherapy: Theory and Technique.* 3rd ed. St. James City, FL: Pine Island Publishers, Inc., 2003.

Bolton, Brett, compiler, editor. *An Edgar Cayce Encyclopedia of Foods for Health and Healing.* Virginia Beach, VA: A.R.E. Press, 1997.

Boyle, Wade, ND, and André Saine, ND. *Lectures in Naturopathic Hydrotherapy.* East Palestine, OH: Buckeye Naturopathic Press, 1991.

Buchman, Dian Dincin. *The Complete Book of Water Therapy.* New Canaan, CT: Keats Publishing, Inc., 1994.

Chaitow, Leon. *Hydrotherapy: Water Therapy for Health and Beauty.* Shaftesbury, Dorset, UK: Element Books Limited, 1999.

Duggan, Joseph, and Sandra Duggan, RN. *Edgar Cayce's Massage, Hydrotherapy and Healing Oils.* Virginia Beach, VA: Inner Vision Publishing Co., 1989.

Edgar Cayce Products: Thirty Years of Research (Virginia Beach, VA: Heritage Publications): 142–143.

Gabbay, Simone. *Nourishing the Body Temple: Edgar Cayce's Approach to Nutrition.* Virginia Beach, VA: A.R.E. Press, 1999.

Grady, Harvey. "A Gift on the Doorstep: The Cayce Impedance Device," *Venture Inward* (Vol. 5, No. 3), May/June 1989: 12–15.

———. "Castor Oil Packs: Scientific Tests Verify Therapeutic Value," *Venture Inward* (Vol. 4, No. 4), July/August 1988: 12–15.

Hanson, Maybritt. "The Wet–Cell: Overcoming MS." *Venture Inward* (Vol. 9, No. 4), July/August 1993: 12–13, 45.

Karp, Reba Ann. *Edgar Cayce Encyclopedia of Healing.* New York: Warner Books, 1986.

Kellogg, John Harvey, MD. *Rational Hydrotherapy.* Battle Creek, MI: Modern Medicine Publishing Company, 1923.

Kneipp, Sebastian. *My Water-Cure.* Translated from the 62nd German edition. Kempten (Bavaria): Joseph Koesel, Publisher, 1897. (Reproduced by Mukelumne Hill, CA: Health Research, 1956)

Kukor, David E. *The Miracle Oil: Secrets of Edgar Cayce's Palma Christi Revealed.* Virginia Beach, VA: A.R.E. Press, 2008.

Lamppa, Ryan. "Ice Massage: The Cold Treatment." *Massage* magazine (January/February 1991), No. 29: 48–50.

McGarey, William A., MD. "The Charred Oak Keg." *Venture Inward* (Vol. 8, No. 4), July/August 1992: 39.

———. *The Edgar Cayce Remedies.* New York: Bantam Books, Inc., 1983.

———. *The Oil That Heals: A Physician's Successes with Castor Oil Treatments.* Virginia Beach, VA: A.R.E. Press, 1994.

———. *Physician's Reference Notebook.* Virginia Beach, VA: A.R.E. Press, 1999.

Nikola, R.J., LMT. *Creatures of Water: Hydrotherapy Textbook.* Salt Lake City: Europa Therapeutic, LLC, 1995.

O'Shea, Michael. "When Do I Use Cold for Injuries, and When Do I Use Heat?" *Parade Magazine,* August 18, 2002: 14.

O'Rourke, Maureen. *Hydrotherapy and Heliotherapy: Natural Healing with Water, Herbs & Sunlight*. Miami, FL: Educating Hands, Inc., 1995.

Parisen, Barbara and Brent. "Our Experiences with the Radio–Active Appliance," *The A.R.E. Journal* (Vol. 13, No. 2), March 1978: 63–69.

Priessnitz, Vincent. *Cold Water Cure*. London: William Strange and E. Smith, 1843. (Reprinted by Health Research, 1976)

Reilly, Harold J., DPhT, DS, and Ruth Hagy Brod. *The Edgar Cayce Handbook for Health Through Drugless Therapy*. 3d ed. Virginia Beach, VA: A.R.E. Press, 2008.

Schlossberg, Brand. "Boost Client Comfort with Heat and Cold Therapy," *Massage Magazine: Buyers Guide 2009*: 138–139.

Schwartzreport, "Issues in Consciousness," Virginia Beach, VA: A.R.E. Conference, November 2–5, 2006.

Taylor, Deborah Seymour. "The Wet–Cell Appliance," *Venture Inward* (Vol. 9, No. 4), July/August 1993: 10–12.

Thrash, Agatha, MD, and Calvin Thrash, MD. *Home Remedies: Hydrotherapy, Massage, Charcoal, and Other Simple Treatments*. Seale, AL: Thrash Publications, 1981.

Turner, Gladys Davis. *An Edgar Cayce Home Medicine Guide*. Virginia Beach, VA: A.R.E. Press, 1983.

Turner, Gladys Davis, and Mae Gimbert St. Clair, eds. *Individual Reference File*. Virginia Beach, VA: A.R.E. Press, 1976.

Who Was Edgar Cayce?
Twentieth Century Psychic and Medical Clairvoyant

Edgar Cayce (pronounced Kay-Cee, 1877-1945) has been called the "sleeping prophet," the "father of holistic medicine," and the most-documented psychic of the 20th century. For more than 40 years of his adult life, Cayce gave psychic "readings" to thousands of seekers while in an unconscious state, diagnosing illnesses and revealing lives lived in the past and prophecies yet to come. But who, exactly, was Edgar Cayce?

Cayce was born on a farm in Hopkinsville, Kentucky, in 1877, and his psychic abilities began to appear as early as his childhood. He was able to see and talk to his late grandfather's spirit, and often played with "imaginary friends" whom he said were spirits on the other side. He also displayed an uncanny ability to memorize the pages of a book simply by sleeping on it. These gifts labeled the young Cayce as strange, but all Cayce really wanted was to help others, especially children.

Later in life, Cayce would find that he had the ability to put himself into a sleep-like state by lying down on a couch, closing his eyes, and folding his hands over his stomach. In this state of relaxation and meditation, he was able to place his mind in contact with all time and space—the universal consciousness, also known as the super-conscious mind. From there, he could respond to questions as broad as, "What are the secrets of the universe?" and "What is my purpose in life?" to as specific as, "What can I do to help my arthritis?" and "How were the pyramids of Egypt built?" His responses to these questions came to be called "readings," and their insights offer practical help and advice to individuals even today.

The majority of Edgar Cayce's readings deal with holistic health and the treatment of illness. Yet, although best known for this material, the sleeping Cayce did not seem to be limited to concerns about the physical body. In fact, in their entirety, the readings discuss an astonishing 10,000 different topics. This vast array of subject matter can be narrowed down into a smaller group of topics that, when compiled together, deal with the following five categories: (1) Health-Related Information; (2) Philosophy and Reincarnation; (3) Dreams and Dream Interpretation; (4) ESP and Psychic Phenomena; and (5) Spiritual Growth, Meditation, and Prayer.

Learn more at EdgarCayce.org.

What Is A.R.E.?

Edgar Cayce founded the non-profit Association for Research and Enlightenment (A.R.E.) in 1931, to explore spirituality, holistic health, intuition, dream interpretation, psychic development, reincarnation, and ancient mysteries—all subjects that frequently came up in the more than 14,000 documented psychic readings given by Cayce.

The Mission of the A.R.E. is to help people transform their lives for the better, through research, education, and application of core concepts found in the Edgar Cayce readings and kindred materials that seek to manifest the love of God and all people and promote the purposefulness of life, the oneness of God, the spiritual nature of humankind, and the connection of body, mind, and spirit.

With an international headquarters in Virginia Beach, Va., a regional headquarters in Houston, regional representatives throughout the U.S., Edgar Cayce Centers in more than thirty countries, and individual members in more than seventy countries, the A.R.E. community is a global network of individuals.

A.R.E. conferences, international tours, camps for children and adults, regional activities, and study groups allow like-minded people to gather for educational and fellowship opportunities worldwide.

A.R.E. offers membership benefits and services that include a quarterly body-mind-spirit member magazine, *Venture Inward*, a member newsletter covering the major topics of the readings, and access to the entire set of readings in an exclusive online database.

Learn more at EdgarCayce.org.

EDGARCAYCE.ORG

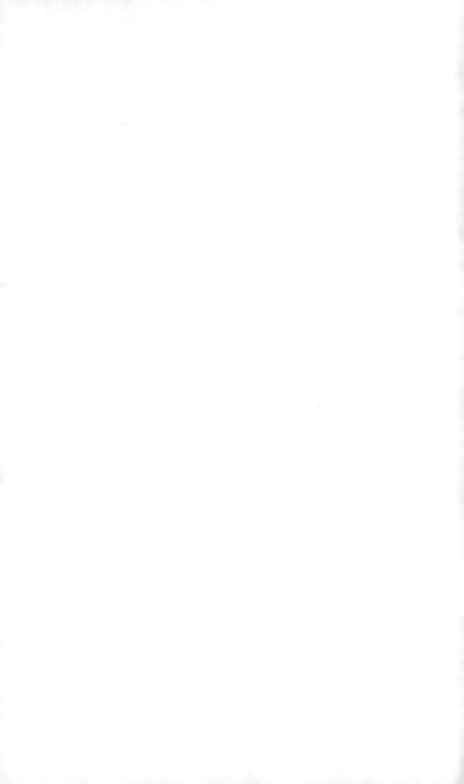